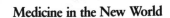

Medicine in the New World

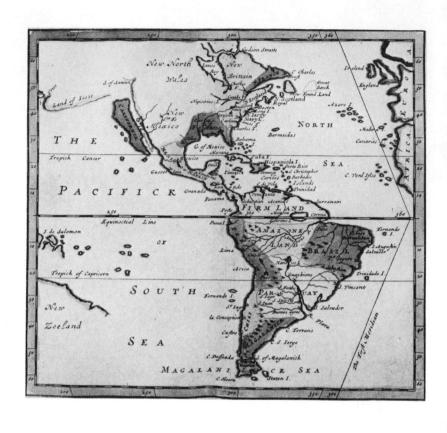

Medicine in the New World

New Spain, New France, and New England

EDITED BY
RONALD L. NUMBERS

THE UNIVERSITY OF TENNESSEE PRESS / KNOXVILLE

Frontispiece: Early map of America showing the location of New
France, New England, and New Spain. From Hermann Moll,
*Atlas Manuale; or, A New Sett [sic] of Maps of All Parts of the
Earth* . . . (London: Printed for J. Churchill and T. Childe, 1713).
Courtesy of the State Historical Society of Wisconsin.

The paper used in this book meets the minimum requirements of the
American National Standard for Permanence of Paper for Printed
Library Materials, Z39.48-1984. Binding materials have been chosen
for durability.

Library of Congress Cataloging-in-Publication Data

Medicine in the New World.

Consists of papers which represent expanded versions of abstracts presented
at session held in conjunction with the 27th International Congress of the
History of Medicine, held in Barcelona, Spain, in 1980.
Bibliography: p.
Includes index.
1. Medicine—Mexico—History—16th century—Congresses. 2. Medicine—
Québec (Province)—History—17th century—Congresses. 3. Medicine—Québec
(Province)—History—18th century—Congresses. 4. Medicine—New England—
History—17th century—Congresses. 5. Medicine—New England—History
18th century—Congresses. I. Numbers, Ronald L. II. International Con-
gress of the History of Medicine (27th : 1980 : Barcelona, Spain) [DNLM: 1.
History of Medicine, 16th Cent.—Mexico—congresses. 2. History of
Medicine, 17th Cent.—New England—congresses. 3. History of Medicine,
17th Cent.—Québec—congresses. 4. History of Medicine, 18th Cent.—New
England—congresses. 5. History of Medicine, 18th Cent.—Québec—
congresses. WZ 56 M4893]
R465.M43 1987   362.1'091812   86-16067
ISBN 0-87049-517-8 (alk. paper)

Contents

Illustrations

Introduction

Ronald L. Numbers

In 1893 a young Wisconsin historian, Frederick Jackson Turner, excited the historical world with an iconoclastic paper on "The Significance of the Frontier in American History." In reaction to the historical dogma that traced American institutions back to imagined roots in Europe, he described American history as "a steady movement away from the influence of Europe" as frontier conditions forced Americans to forsake the rigid intellectual systems and social arrangements of the Old World in favor of a democratic and individualistic way of life.[1]

Turner's novel frontier thesis captured the imagination of generations of American historians, eager to celebrate their country's distinctiveness. Although a few scholars, such as the legal historian Julius Goebel, Jr., dismissed it as "an artificial and labored explanation" that overlooked important similarities between practices in rural England and in the colonies, the frontier hypothesis — and environmentalist theories in general — remained in historiographical fashion for decades.[2] Richard B. Morris credited the frontier with liberating American law from "many of the shackles of English medievalism"; Sidney E. Mead invoked "the subtle magic of the new land" to explain the "Americanization" of Christianity; Malcolm Sydney Beinfield argued that the "rugged environment" of colonial New England not only erased the traditional distinctions separating physicians, surgeons, and apothecaries, but also encouraged colonists to replace Old World therapies with home-made herbals.[3] John W. Oliver, though aware that much of colonial technology had simply been transplanted from the Old World, nevertheless maintained that the "new environment" and "Yankee ingenuity" had promoted technological innovation. I. Bernard Cohen in 1941 attributed Benjamin Franklin's discoveries in electricity, the New World's most stunning scientific achievement, to his virtual ignorance of European physics—although fifteen years later he reversed himself and rejected as "romantic" the notion that Franklin could have made his discoveries in an intellectual vacuum.[4]

The most eloquent and comprehensive attempt to explain the rise of a distinctive American civilization in environmentalist terms appeared in Daniel J. Boorstin's study *The Americans: The Colonial Experience* (1958). According to Boorstin, the primitive conditions that greeted settlers from the Old World forced them to ditch the "cumbersome cultural baggage" they had brought from home and turned them into a practical, nontheoretical people who learned from experience, not books. Their schools trained generalists rather than specialists, and their ministers preached homilies rather than systematic theology. Their lawyers were "unspecialized"; their soldiers, "unprofessional." Making a virtue of ignorance, Boorstin argued that Franklin's discovery "illustrated the triumph of naïveté over learning" and showed that "an American could discover something, even in physics, simply because he was less learned than his European colleagues." In discussing medicine, he alleged that the New World environment had fused the English "specialities" of medicine, surgery, and pharmacy into a distinctively American healer: the general practitioner. And because these doctors escaped the contaminating influence of European academic medicine by learning at the bedside rather than in the lecture hall, they approached healing empirically and open-mindedly. The beneficiary of this was the colonial patient—"lucky that so much learned error had not been brought to these shores."[5]

During the late 1950s the environmentalist interpretation of colonial American history reached its crest. In addition to Boorstin's book, there appeared a collection of essays, edited by James Morton Smith, that focused on the manner in which the American wilderness transformed English institutions in the seventeenth century. As one of the contributors, Oscar Handlin, observed, the Europeans who settled the New World "pitched upon the edge

of an almost empty continent; and the existence of open space
to which men could withdraw remained a constant condition of
their life," loosening the bonds that had previously kept the social
structure intact. A year later Bernard Bailyn brought out his much-
debated analysis of *Education in the Forming of American Society,* in which he, too, stressed "the rapid breakdown of traditional European society in its wilderness setting." The New World
experience, he argued, eroded the family's traditional role in trans-
mitting culture to the young. Threatened by the prospect of slip-
ping into "barbarism," colonial Americans turned to schools to
educate their youth.[6]

Before long, however, a reaction to such unrestrained environ-
mentalism set in, prompted in part by a growing uneasiness about
America's claim to uniqueness, an awareness that comparative studies did not support many of the assertions of the frontier school,
and the appearance in the 1960s and 1970s of several influential
analyses of New England towns.[7] Turner himself had pointedly re-
frained from looking at the French and Spanish frontier in the New
World, and few of his disciples had taken the time to acquaint themselves with European or non-English colonial history.[8] In 1966
David J. Rothman publicly chastized Bailyn and others for their neglect of European social history, which he claimed had led them to
exaggerate the effects of "the American wilderness" on the colonial
family. Kenneth A. Lockridge in an innovative study of *Literacy
in Colonial New England* (1974), which in passing compared the
New England experience with that of the Scots and the Swedes,
also took Bailyn and the environmentalists to task for insisting
that the wilderness had spurred the growth of schools and the
spread of literacy. If anything, he argued, the frontier conditions
of seventeenth-century New England had proved a "handicap."
Protestantism, not the wilderness, had promoted literacy.[9]

Perhaps the most scathing indictment of the environmentalists
appeared in Michael Kammen's *People of Paradox: An Inquiry
Concerning the Origins of American Civilization* (1972), which
examined the colonial experience in comparative perspective. "Historians who have been inoculated with the serum of environmen-
talism, from Turner to Boorstin," he wrote,

> have reacted virulently to any suggestion that things European
> might long survive the trans-Atlantic voyage to North America. Yet

the *peculiarly* transforming powers of oceans, forests, and plains located between 32 and 48 degrees of latitude are difficult to discover.
. . . Since the civilizations of North and South America have evolved in such profoundly dissimilar ways, it is difficult to determine just what the *unique* role of environment has been in the history of these United States.

Although Kammen stopped short of denying any influence to the environment, he emphasized that "once the earliest settlements were established, essentially by mid-seventeenth century, provincial culture in significant ways 'began to line up again with English traditions.'" Addressing the by-now trite argument that New World societies could not have maintained the complex professional arrangements of the Old World, including the several medical guilds, he noted that "the professions were not so highly developed in Stuart and Hanoverian England as we have assumed; nor were they so primitive in provincial America as some had suspected."[10]

A host of specialized studies that began appearing in the 1960s lent credence to Kammen's contention. T.H. Breen, for example, traced the localism characteristic of New England society, long thought to be a New World development, back to the colonists' opposition to centralization in Old England. George L. Haskins followed Goebel in emphasizing the similarities between the legal practices of rural England and those of colonial Massachusetts. And, in reply to Mead's suggestion that the New World had prompted a "shift from a 'sacerdotal' to an 'evangelical' type of ministry," David D. Hall maintained that an evangelical understanding of the ministry, far from being the "consequence of Americanization," was in fact an English import. In surveys of American religious history Sidney E. Ahlstrom and Winthrop S. Hudson also parted ways with Mead. "After a long period in which historians have emphasized the uniqueness of almost everything American," wrote Hudson, "it is becoming increasingly clear that the United States can properly be understood only as an integral part of a larger European society."[11]

Such statements did not, of course, rule out the possibility of distinctive developments in the New World, even ones caused specifically by the environment. As Robert M. Kingdon pointed out in an essay comparing Protestant churches in Geneva and Boston, colonial Americans tended to create parishes based on "common ideas or social attachments" rather than on place of residence, which was typical of Europe, where established churches often held monopolies. And as Brooke Hindle observed, because of the relative abundance of wood in the New World, the material culture of the colonies took on a distinctively "American" appearance. Although not prone to environmentalist explanations—he at times blamed the American environment for inhibiting the growth of science and stressed the dependence upon Britain in the transfer of technology to the colonies—Hindle believed that the "ubiquity of wood in the American scene and the relative ease of working it encouraged both technological change and personal, occupational mobility."[12] Nevertheless, with few exceptions, environmental determinism and appeals to the frontier fell out of favor with American historians. In a major reappraisal of the colonial experience that grew out of a conference organized in 1981 by Jack P. Greene and J.R. Pole, the editors pointed out that only one of the fourteen contributors had "a good word to say for the concept of American exceptionalism."[13]

Among historians of medicine, Richard Harrison Shryock led the effort to correct the prevailing view "that English professional distinctions broke down or were deliberately abandoned in the presence of the American environment." It was fallacious, he wrote in *Medicine and Society in America, 1660–1860* (1960), to contrast colonial medical practice with that of London, since most English immigrants came from rural areas and small towns, where medical men commonly combined the practice of internal medicine with surgery and pharmacy. English physicians, like the upper classes generally, seldom sought a new life on the American frontier:

> Hence the story here was partially one of selective immigration rather than simply of adaptation to environment. There was no rejection of London distinctions in principle, nor was any new, native type of practice set up. All that happened was that few of the upper stratum of medical men came over, and that persons behaving like British apothecaries (general practitioners) found themselves in consequence the sole colonial profession.

In a brief, virtually unprecedented, comparison, he pointed out that the experience of New Spain, which regulated medicine in

Old World fashion, contradicted the notion that medical practice could not be controlled in a new society.[14]

Other medical historians soon followed Shryock in highlighting the continuities rather than the discontinuities between medical practice in the Old and New Worlds. Joseph F. Kett and, less directly, Whitfield J. Bell, Jr. repeated Shryock's warning against attaching too much significance to the general practice of colonial doctors because, as Kett pointed out, even within London, to say nothing of provincial England, the roles of physician, surgeon, and apothecary had begun to merge. In a succinct appraisal of "Medical Colonization of the New World," published in 1963, Francisco Guerra concluded that "it was the European and not the indigenous element which dominated the shaping of medicine in the American continent during the years of colonization."[15]

Despite such attacks on the environmentalist interpretation of colonial medical history, echoes of Turner and Boorstin have continued to reverberate through the literature on American medicine, especially in general surveys, down to the present. For example, in *The Healers: The Rise of the Medical Establishment* (1976) John Duffy appeals to "frontier conditions and the fluidity of American society" to explain the absence of distinctions between physicians and surgeons in the colonies; and Lester S. King, in *American Medicine Comes of Age, 1840–1920* (1984), argues that the New World "environment differed so markedly from that of Great Britain that the institutions suitable for the mother country were no longer adaptive to the new conditions." Referring to the hierarchical division of medicine purportedly found in England, he asserts that "the social setting in America would not accept a blatant division into a medical aristocracy and a residual class with lower status." Even Paul Starr, in his prize-winning study of *The Social Transformation of American Medicine* (1982), invokes an American aversion to class distinctions (as well as selective migration) to explain the presumed differences between the hierarchical English arrangement and the democratic practice of medicine found in America.[16]

The persistence of such contradictory opinions regarding what may well be the central issue in the history of early American health care suggests the need for a systematic inquiry into the relationship between Old and New World medicine. Our task in this volume is two-fold. First, to assess the extent to which medicine was transformed in its journey to the New World, we must mine what practices prevailed in the Old—and not just in the capitals of Europe but in the countryside as well. Only in this way can we avoid the hazard of mistakenly attributing novelty to New World arrangements out of ignorance of Old World customs. Second, to identify what was possible in a New World environment, we need to compare experiences in various parts of the Americas, bearing in mind, of course, that no two settings were identical. This two-pronged approach allows us to engage in what one historian has called "a primitive form of historical 'experimentation.'"[17]

In the essays that follow, three medical historians, each familiar with developments on both sides of the Atlantic, survey respectively the transit of medical institutions and practices from Spain to New Spain (present-day Mexico), from France to New France (particularly the province of Quebec), and from England to New England (the northeastern United States). These parallel accounts, though focusing on slightly different time frames the sixteenth century for New Spain, the seventeenth and eighteenth centuries for New France and New England—provide the basis for a concluding analysis of New World medical history based on both trans Atlantic and trans-colonial comparisons.

This volume originated with a session on "Medicine in the New World" held in conjunction with the XXVIIth International Congress of the History of Medicine in Barcelona, Spain, in the summer of 1980. On that occasion the four contributors to this volume each read brief summaries of their findings, which subsequently appeared in the *Actas* of the Congress.[18] The essays that appear in the present volume represent a ten- to fifteen-fold expansion of these previously published abstracts. We are grateful to Carolyn Hackler, of the Department of the History of Medicine at the University of Wisconsin-Madison, for typing the final manuscript.

NOTES

I would like to thank Charlotte Borst for her bibliographic assistance in the preparation of this introduction.

1. Frederick Jackson Turner, *The Frontier in American History* (New York: Henry Holt, 1920), 4. This collection of essays includes "The

Significance of the Frontier in American History," first published in 1893.

2. Julius Goebel, Jr., "King's Law and Local Custom in Seventeenth Century New England," *Columbia Law Review* (1931), *31:*420, 448. See also Goebel's later essay, "Law Enforcement in Colonial New York: An Introduction," in *Essays in the History of Early American Law,* ed. David H. Flaherty (Chapel Hill: Univ. of North Carolina Press, 1969), 367–91, in which he blames Roscoe Pound for applying Turner's theory to the history of early American law.

3. Richard B. Morris, *Studies in the History of American Law: With Special Reference to the 17th and 18th Centuries,* vol. 316 of *Columbia Studies in History* (New York: Columbia Univ. Press, 1930), 17–20, 41–42, 46; Sidney E. Mead, "The Rise of the Evangelical Conception of the Ministry in America (1607–1850)," in *The Ministry in Historical Perspective,* ed. H. Richard Niebuhr and Daniel D. Williams (New York: Harper & Brothers, 1956), 208; Malcolm Sydney Beinfield, "The Early New England Doctor: An Adaptation to a Provincial Environment," *Yale Journal of Biology and Medicine* (1942–43), *15:*99–132, 271–88. Mead's mentor, William Warren Sweet, also emphasized the frontier experience and "the Americanization of Christianity"; see, e.g., his *The Story of Religion in America* (New York: Harper & Brothers, 1930) and *Religion in Colonial America* (New York: Scribner's, 1942), as well as James L. Ash, Jr., *Protestantism and the American University: An Intellectual Biography of William Warren Sweet* (Dallas: Southern Methodist Univ. Press, 1982), 44–48.

4. John W. Oliver, *History of American Technology* (New York: Ronald Press, 1956), pt. I; I. Bernard Cohen, *Benjamin Franklin's Experiments* (Cambridge, Mass.: Harvard Univ. Press, 1941); I. Bernard Cohen, *Franklin and Newton: An Inquiry into Speculative Newtonian Experimental Science and Franklin's Work in Electricity as an Example Thereof* (Philadelphia: American Philosophical Society, 1956).

5. Daniel J. Boorstin, *The Americans: The Colonial Experience* (New York: Random House, 1958), 149, 208–39, 251–52. In *Science in the British Colonies of America* (Urbana: Univ. of Illinois Press, 1970), 640–42, Raymond Phineas Stearns rejects Cohen's claim in *Franklin and Newton* that Franklin was working within the context of European science in favor of Boorstin's interpretation of Franklin's achievement.

6. Oscar Handlin, "The Significance of the Seventeenth Century," in *Seventeenth-Century America: Essays in Colonial History,* ed. James Morton Smith (Chapel Hill: Univ. of North Carolina Press, 1959), 3–12; Bernard Bailyn, *Education in the Forming of American Society: Needs and Opportunities for Study* (1960; rpt. New York: Norton, 1972), 17, 73. For a less environmentalistic interpretation than Bailyn's, see Lawrence

A. Cremin, *American Education: The Colonial Experience, 1607–1783* (New York: Harper & Row, 1970).

7. For an introduction to the pioneering work of such historians as Sumner Chilton Powell, John Demos, Philip J. Greven, Jr., and Kenneth Lockridge, see Richard S. Dunn, "The Social History of Early New England," *American Quarterly* (1972), 24:661–79.

8. Turner, *Frontier in American History,* unpaginated preface. On the reaction against Turner's thesis, see, e.g., George M. Fredrickson, "Comparative History," in *The Past before Us: Contemporary Historical Writing in the United States,* ed. Michael Kammen (Ithaca, N.Y.: Cornell Univ. Press, 1980), 462–63.

9. David J. Rothman, "A Note on the Study of the Colonial Family," *William and Mary Quarterly,* 3rd ser. (1966), 23:627–34; Kenneth A. Lockridge, *Literacy in Colonial New England: An Enquiry into the Social Context of Literacy in the Early Modern West* (New York: Norton, 1974), 43–45. In an appendix to the Lockridge book entitled "The Educational Response to the American Wilderness," pp. 103–108, Richard Alterman concluded that "there is no evidence that the wilderness shattered the essentially nuclear families which arrived in America."

10. Michael Kammen, *People of Paradox: An Inquiry Concerning the Origins of American Civilization* (New York: Knopf, 1972), 22–29.

11. T.H. Breen, "Persistent Localism: English Social Change and the Shaping of New England Institutions," *William and Mary Quarterly,* 3rd ser. (1975), 32:3–28; T.H. Breen, "Transfer of Culture: Chance and Design in Shaping Massachusetts Bay, 1630–1660," *New England Historical and Genealogical Register* (1978), 132:3–17; George L. Haskins, "Reception of the Common Law in Seventeenth-Century Massachusetts: A Case Study," in *Law and Authority in Colonial America: Selected Essays,* ed. George Athan Billias (Barre, Mass.: Barre Publishers, 1965), 17–31; David D. Hall, *The Faithful Shepherd: A History of the New England Ministry in the Seventeenth Century* (Chapel Hill: Univ. of North Carolina Press, 1972), ix–xi; Sidney E. Ahlstrom, *A Religious History of the American People* (New Haven: Yale Univ. Press, 1972), 453–54; Winthrop S. Hudson, *Religion in America,* 2nd ed. (New York: Scribner's, 1973), 3. See also David Grayson Allen, *In English Ways: The Movement of Societies and the Transferal of English Local Law and Custom to Massachusetts Bay in the Seventeenth Century* (Chapel Hill: Univ. of North Carolina Press, 1981), which emphasizes "the fundamentally English form and style of New England local institutions in the early seventeenth century" (xv); and Jonathan L. Fairbanks and Robert F. Trent, eds., *New England Begins: The Seventeenth Century,* 3 vols. (Boston: Museum of Fine Arts, 1982), in which Fairbanks contends that "the settlers transferred their entire culture to the New World" (1:xvii).

12. Robert M. Kingdon, "Protestant Parishes in the Old World and the New: The Cases of Geneva and Boston," *Church History* (1979), *48*:290–304; Brooke Hindle, ed., *Material Culture in the Wooden Age* (Tarrytown, N.Y.: Sleepy Hollow Press, 1981), 11; Brooke Hindle, *Technology in Early America: Needs and Opportunities for Study* (Chapel Hill: Univ. of North Carolina Press, 1966), 26, 89. On the role of the environment in inhibiting science, see Brooke Hindle, *The Pursuit of Science in Revolutionary America, 1735–1789* (Chapel Hill: Univ. of North Carolina Press, 1956), 3. Like Hindle, Darrett B. Rutman has tended to stress the cultural baggage the colonists brought with them, while admitting that the environment selected those parts of the baggage "most appropriate to the colonial situation"; see Rutman, *The Morning of America, 1603–1789* (Boston: Houghton Mifflin, 1971), 42–47. G.B. Warden, "Law Reform in England and New England, 1620 to 1660," *William and Mary Quarterly*, 3rd ser. (1978), *35*:668–90, takes a similarly eclectic position with respect to early legal history.

13. Jack P. Greene and J.R. Pole, eds., *Colonial British America: Essays in the New History of the Early Modern Era* (Baltimore: Johns Hopkins Univ. Press, 1984), 10. Exceptions to this generalization include A.L. Burt, "If Turner Had Looked at Canada, Australia, and New Zealand When He Wrote about the West," in *The Frontier in Perspective*, ed. Walker D. Wyman and Clifton B. Kroeber (Madison: Univ. of Wisconsin Press, 1965), 59–77; and Ray Allen Billington, "Frontiers," in *The Comparative Approach to American History*, ed. C. Vann Woodward (New York: Basic Books, 1968), 75–90.

14. Richard Harrison Shryock, *Medicine and Society in America, 1660–1860* (New York: New York Univ. Press, 1960), 3–12. See also Shryock, *Medical Licensing in America, 1650–1965* (Baltimore: Johns Hopkins Press, 1967), 8–9.

15. Joseph F. Kett, "Provincial Medical Practice in England, 1730–1815," *Journal of the History of Medicine and Allied Sciences* (1964), *19*:17–29; Kett, *The Formation of the American Medical Profession: The Role of Institutions, 1780–1860* (New Haven: Yale Univ. Press, 1968), 1–6; Whitfield J. Bell, Jr., "A Portrait of the Colonial Physician," *Bulletin of the History of Medicine* (1970), *44*:499, 501; Francisco Guerra, "Medical Colonization of the New World," *Medical History* (1963) *7*:147–54. See also Toby Gelfand, "The Origins of a Modern Concept of Medical Specialization: John Morgan's *Discourse* of 1765," *Bulletin of the History of Medicine* (1976), *50*:511–35; and Ivan Waddington, *The Medical Profession in the Industrial Revolution* (Dublin: Gill and Macmillan, 1984), 181–96.

16. John Duffy, *The Healers: The Rise of the Medical Establishment* (New York: McGraw-Hill, 1976), 24–25; Lester S. King, *American Medi-

cine Comes of Age, 1840–1920 (Chicago: American Medical Association, 1984), 1, 6; Paul Starr, *The Social Transformation of American Medicine* (New York: Basic Books, 1982), 34–40. See also John Duffy, *Epidemics in Colonial America* (Baton Rouge: Louisiana State Univ. Press, 1953), 7. In his survey of "Medical Professionalism" in the *Encyclopedia of Bioethics,* ed. Warren T. Reich, 4 vols. (New York: Free Press, 1978), 3:1030, Martin S. Pernick argues that "The shortage of gentleman-practitioners in the colonies broke down the distinctions among physicians, surgeons, and druggists."

17. Peter Kolchin, "Comparing American History," in *The Promise of American History,* ed. Stanley I. Kutler and Stanley N. Katz (Baltimore: Johns Hopkins Univ. Press, 1982), 65.

18. Guenter B. Risse, "Medicine in New Spain: Institutions and Practice 1570–1621," in *Actas,* XXVII Congreso Internacional de Historia de la Medicina, 2 vols. (Barcelona: Acadèmia de Ciències Mèdiques de Catalunya i Balears, 1981), 1:207–11; Toby Gelfand, "Medicine in New France: Les Francais Look at les Canadiens during the Seven Years' War," ibid., 2:511–16; Ronald L. Numbers, "Medicine in the New World: A Comparison," ibid., 2:592–95. Eric Christianson's abstract did not appear in the proceedings of the Congress.

1

Medicine in New Spain

GUENTER B. RISSE

In the century after Columbus discovered the New World and Cortés conquered the Aztec empire, Spanish immigrants gradually settled in New Spain and organized a society based on Castilian values and institutions. The transfer of medical ideas and institutions began early and shaped the health-care experience of the entire colony. Thus, to understand New World medical events, it is essential first to examine medical developments in Spain during the fifteenth and sixteenth centuries.[1]

MEDICINE IN SPAIN

Spain's "golden age" spanned the period between the new monarchy of the "Catholic Kings" (1475) and the death of Philip II in 1598, during which Spaniards discovered and colonized vast territories in the New World and transformed a hitherto politically fragmented country into a formidable world power.[2] Although walled cities dotted the countryside, the vast majority of the eight million inhabitants of Spain lived in rural areas. Spain, like the rest of Europe, was not a healthful place in which to live. According to contemporary reports, the burden of disease had extensive demographic and economic consequences.[3]

Plague, a frequent visitor since the mid-fourteenth century, usually struck the coastal Spanish cities located on the shores of the

Mediterranean Sea and then spread in a southwesterly direction into Catalonia and Andalucía. In the late fifteenth century, for example, Mallorca, Barcelona, and Zaragoza all reported multiple outbreaks, while Valencia, Seville, and Granada each suffered through at least one. These periodic visitations continued unabated during the following century, often spreading beyond the coastal strip to the interior.[4] One epidemic alone, in 1596, took an estimated 600,000 lives, representing about 8 percent of the entire Spanish population.

Less destructive, but still significant health problems, were two possibly "new" diseases: typhus and syphilis. The former, popularly termed *tabardillo* or *pintas*, erupted in 1489 among the troops engaged in the war against the Moors and reemerged between 1557 and 1570. Syphilis or *bubas,* as it was commonly known, first appeared in 1495 during the wars in Italy. Initially an affliction of soldiers and prostitutes, this virulent disease rapidly spread to the upper and middle classes of society.[5] Smallpox or *viruelas* also occasionally assumed epidemic proportions in Spain. Leprosy, an endemic medieval scourge already in decline, continued to terrorize the people, afflicting a sizeable number of inhabitants and prompting royal regulations to insure the institutional isolation of those believed to suffer from the disease.

Medical Personnel

Renaissance Spain suffered from a severe shortage of university-trained medical personnel. At the top of the professional pyramid was the physician with a doctoral degree, a rarity limited to those seeking an academic career. Not far below those doctors were the *licenciado* or licentiate and the *bachiller* or bachelor, both of whom held university degrees conferred to candidates who had completed their prescribed medical studies but were unwilling or financially unable to undergo the multiple formalities required for the doctorate.[6]

One step further down in the medical hierarchy were the so-called Latin surgeons, a distinct but growing minority of surgeons with university training. The University of Valencia established a chair of surgery as early as 1509, but the University of Salamanca did not do so until 1566. Both physicians and Latin surgeons practiced mostly in Spanish cities and at the royal court.

They were often employed by municipalities or hospitals and some-times formed part of the retinues of nobles and prominent clergy.

Most Spanish surgeons during the sixteenth century were Ro-mance surgeons, that is, individuals without university education who had received their often meager training entirely by appren-ticeship. To provide them with a minimum of systematized knowl-edge, authors of surgical textbooks often wrote in the vernacular. Many Romance surgeons found employment in the expanding armies and navies of the empire.

The shortage of trained health professionals can be glimpsed from fragmentary evidence gathered in Valencia, a major urban center. In 1400, for example, records indicate the presence in the city of only nineteen physicians and eight surgeons for a popula-tion of about 30,000, a ratio that remained constant for the next two centuries and was actually the highest in the Iberian penin-sula.[7] To fill the large void in health care created by so small a number of physicians and surgeons, both aristocrats and the gen-eral public often had recourse to "empirics" who treated specific problems demanding practical skills: the *algebrista* or bone set-ter, who reduced dislocations and set fractures; the *hernista*, who reduced and managed hernias; the *sacador de la piedra*, who re-moved painful bladder stones; the *batidor de la catarata*, who couched cataracts; the *sacamuelas*, who extracted teeth; and the popular midwife, variously called *comadre, madrina* or *partera*.[8] Magical healers, including astrologers and necromantic conjur-ers, were especially popular with the masses.

The shortage of qualified health professionals in sixteenth-cen-tury Spain was aggravated by governmental policies toward the Jewish and Morisco minorities. In late medieval times Jews and Moors had almost monopolized the medical profession; they oc-cupied prominent posts at the royal court, took care of clergymen, and worked as municipal physicians. The expulsion of the Jews, decreed in 1492 by the Catholic Kings, was followed in 1501 with the requirement of blood purity or *limpieza de sangre* for persons desiring to practice medicine. The exclusion of healers of Jewish ancestry created considerable problems for a number of municipalities.[9]

The atmosphere of racial and religious intolerance that gripped Spain, especially during the late-sixteenth-century Counter Ref-ormation, resulted in restrictions that barred Moors and Moriscos

(Moorish converts to Catholicism) from universities and prohibited them from legally practicing medicine. The concerted efforts of the Catholic majority, motivated by racial and economic considerations, forced Morisco healers into an illegal and marginal status. The harrassment of Morisco practitioners, including prohibiting midwives from practicing in Granada and Valencia, culminated with their physical banishment from Spain, decreed in 1609.[10]

During the fifteenth and sixteenth centuries Spain regulated medical activities more intensively than any other European country. Since the Middle Ages various Spanish authorities had examined physicians and surgeons, and in 1420 Alfonso V of Aragón established a tribunal to screen out incompetent practitioners. Composed of two physicians and two surgeons, this body checked credentials, conducted examinations, and issued licenses. Because the king's personal physician, the *protomédico* or first physician, served on this tribunal, it eventually came to be called the *protomedicato*.[11]

In 1477, following the country's unification, the rulers created a central *protomedicato* empowered to examine not only physicians, surgeons, and midwives, but also apothecaries, spice merchants, and their wares. They also expanded the body's licensing functions to include judicial responsibilities. By the sixteenth century the *protomedicato* included physicians, auditors, magistrates, a judge, and several law enforcement agents. Surgeons and apothecaries were required to have a minimum of four years of training as apprentices before becoming eligible for examination, and even physicians with medical degrees had to demonstrate their diagnostic and therapeutic skills with hospitalized patients. Licenses were issued upon successful passage of the examination and the payment of fees.[12]

In 1567, under Philip II, midwives and grocers dealing in spices and aromatic drugs were excluded from the *protomedicato's* jurisdiction, and in 1588 the king authorized specific licenses for empirical healers such as those who set bones, couched cataracts, removed bladder stones, and reduced hernias. These persons, however, were only allowed to carry out their activities in consultation with licensed surgeons. Still later, Philip III in 1603 legalized the activities of Romance surgeons, provided they could demonstrate a background of five years in practice, two while apprenticed to a physician or master surgeon and three working in a hospital. These new regulations suggest that the authorities wished to expand the scope of legalized medical practice to meet severe shortages produced in part by immigration to the New World and the exclusion of Jewish and Morisco healers.

Subsequent developments in the early seventeenth century expanded the executive and judicial functions of the *protomedicato*. In addition to granting practicing privileges, inspecting drugstores and food-producing establishments, and prosecuting violators, the institution now assumed the task of enforcing quarantines, segregating contagious patients, and monitoring the conditions of buildings, plazas, streets, hospitals, and cemeteries during epidemics. The prosecution of *curanderos,* that is, irregular self-appointed healers, was often taken over by the Inquisition in cases involving magico-religious cures or Morisco or Jewish healers.

Medical Education

The panorama of Spanish medical education during the fifteenth and sixteenth centuries reveals a highly formalized system of theoretical instruction, modeled on the curriculum of the University of Salamanca, which began training physicians in 1252. During the sixteenth century, Spain considerably expanded its university system as royalty, religious orders, and city authorities vied for the privilege of granting degrees. Medical education became available at a number of institutions, such as the University of Valencia (1500), Zaragoza (1500), Seville (1508), and especially Alcalá de Henares (1510), which quickly became, with Salamanca and Valladolid, one of the most famous institutions of higher learning in Spain. Alcalá trained the bulk of physicians who formed the professional elite in New Spain after 1570.[13]

Medical education at Alcalá and elsewhere was purely theoretical. Moreover, in contrast to the more populous Salamanca with its Hospital de Santa Maria la Blanca, Alcalá lacked any clinical facilities whatsoever. According to its 1510 regulations, the university closely followed the Salamanca model, establishing two chairs of medicine named in accordance with canonical hours: *prima* (morning) and *vísperas* (vesper). In most institutions the *prima* chair was considered to be the primary or original chair, affording its holder higher prestige and salary than other professors.[14]

In 1530, Salamanca added a *tercera* or third chair to its curriculum. A chair of anatomy followed in 1551, and a fifth faculty position, in surgery, was created in 1556. During the last third of the sixteenth century Alcalá also expanded its academic staff, establishing two additional chairs of *prima* and *vísperas*. A fifth chair, of surgery, was created in 1594 to facilitate the training of Latin surgeons and provide physicians with greater surgical knowledge. One of Alcalá's *vísperas* professors taught anatomy, facilitated by a royal provision of 4 April 1559 that allowed the dissection of executed criminals and persons who had died in hospitals. Spain had a strong tradition of anatomical dissection, dating back at least to 1488, when King Ferdinand gave the medico-surgical *cofradía* of Saints Cosmas and Damian in Zaragoza permission to dissect dead inmates from the local Hospital de Santa María de Gracia.

Curricular reforms during the sixteenth century amounted to little more than substituting the expurgated classics of Hippocrates and Galen for readings from Avicenna. Perhaps the greatest innovation was the previously mentioned establishment of surgical chairs, first at Salamanca (1556) and later Alcalá (1594) and Valladolid (1594). The meshing of medical and surgical education equipped graduates who immigrated to the New World with the skills needed to face the tasks awaiting them across the Atlantic.[15]

To begin the academic study of medicine in Spain a candidate needed to possess a bachelor's degree in arts, acquired after four years of university study.[16] The four-year medical curriculum was based on lectures and commentaries on the writings of various ancient and medieval authorities.[17] Professors lectured for exactly one hour daily. Half of that time they dictated in Latin from a text in front of them; the remainder of the hour they explained and interpreted the quoted text, occasionally in the vernacular. Teachers were also required to hold less formal question-and-answer sessions outside the classrooms; these were called *al poste*, next to the pillar. All academics were prohibited from teaching in their houses and from giving private lessons.

At the conclusion of the four years, students had to serve a six-month practical apprenticeship with a faculty member before receiving their bachelor of medicine diploma. This clinical externship, designed to balance the purely theoretical instruction, was extended in 1563 to two years. With a bachelor of medicine degree in hand, physicians became eligible for licensing, which allowed them to practice medicine. The newly graduated physician, however, still had to be examined by local and later royal *proto-medicatos,* a sometimes humiliating experience that seriously encroached upon the powers of the universities and thus became a perennial source of conflict. To obtain a licenciate in medicine in the sixteenth century, physicians holding a bachelor of medicine degree had to continue in residence for another three years, reading further from the works of Avicenna, Hippocrates, and Galen. At the end of each year, the candidates were publicly examined in a ceremony called *primer principio* (first year), *segundo principio* (second year), and *tercer principio* (third year). The last examination was a rigorous pass-or-fail test, administered by the dean and no more than twelve faculty members.[18]

Students passing the *tercer principio* faced two more examinations: the *quolibeto* and *Alfonsina*. The former was another critical pass-or-fail test; the latter, a solemn public examination, where the candidate displayed his knowledge and rhetorical skills in front of the medical and arts faculties. Topics for the *Alfonsina* examination were selected twenty hours in advance by using the *tres puntos* (three points) system, which consisted of using a pointed instrument to select at random passages from the writings of Galen or Avicenna. The candidate then chose one of these selections as the basis of his speech and discussion.[19]

After successfully completing this requirement, future licenciates were subjected to the *información,* a formal interrogation in the presence of the rector and secretary of the university concerning their Catholic orthodoxy and *limpieza de sangre.* Then came the *paraninfo* or harbinger of good news, a festive ceremony in church during which an emissary officially announced the imminent granting of their degrees. The following day university officials and faculty returned to the church to vote on the *rótulo,* a ranked list of candidates that determined the order in which diplomas were awarded. The *rótulo* or honor roll was a constant source of petty rivalries and internecine feuds. At Alcalá the practice was occasionally abandoned in the sixteenth century, only to return because of the need for distinguishing excellence: the higher ranked *licenciados* had priority in receiving doctorates. [20]

Although the licenciate in medicine was more than adequate for practicing medicine, it did not entitle holders to compete for academic positions, which required a doctorate degree. The formalities associated with acquiring an M.D., which apparently required no additional study, involved a great deal of additional expense. Once the candidate was accepted for the high degree, he went through an elaborate sequence of ceremonies divided into two groups: the *víspera* or preliminary activities, and the *borla* (literally the tassel). Beginning the preliminary festivities was another *acto del paraninfo,* announcing the date of graduation, followed by speeches and an examination. Then came the *vejamen* or insulting speech, in which a faculty member jokingly mocked the future doctor and made fun of his frailties, and finally the *paseo,* a ride through town on horseback in the company of university officials and academics.

The *borla* began with the *concurrencia,* in which the nominee, his sponsors, family, and friends assembled in church. The ceremony continued with speeches by two professors named *gallo y gallina*—rooster and hen—who "cackled" on the virtues of the candidate. Then the new doctor took an oath and received the appropriate insignias and diploma, the crowning act in a ritual displaying much medieval pomp and pageantry.[21]

Between 1570 and 1600, Alcalá graduated 409 bachelors, 91 licenciates, and 81 doctors of medicine. The number of students fluctated widely each year, with the average being about 130.[22]

Medical professors lectured about 225 days a year. Besides their academic obligations, they were required at Alcalá to provide medical care to sick students, friars at the monastery, inmates at the local hospital, and certain of the poor. In the mid-sixteenth century the holder of the *prima chair* received 75,000 *maravedís* per year, an adequate if not generous salary. Fees received for examining degree candidates and awarding diplomas could increase his income to 87,000 *maravedís.*[23]

Hospitals

A vigorous hospital movement began in Spain during the fourteenth and fifteenth centuries, although its roots go back to the Middle Ages. Early hospitals in the Latin West, dating from the sixth to the ninth centuries, stressed hospitality rather than medical care. Most of them were inns, located on roads leading to shrines and cities, often next to monasteries. They ministered to hungry, tired, and ill wayfarers as an expression of Christian charity.[24] Beginning in the eleventh century, a growing population, together with increased trade and travel, created adverse health conditions and promoted disease. To cope with this situation, new monastic orders and lay brotherhoods organized charitable institutions for the specific purpose of taking care of the sick.[25] In 1195, Alfonso VIII founded the Hospital del Rey in Burgos, a city in northern Spain. Barcelona acquired its first hospital, the Hospital de Santa Cruz, in 1229; Valencia erected a general hospital in 1238. The order of Knights of St. Anthony, created in 1214 to care for people afflicted with ergotism, founded hospitals in Mallorca (1230) and Salamanca (1256).

While shifting its emphasis from hospitality to therapy, the medieval hospital remained basically a religious institution, in which prayer, mass, and the administration of sacraments took precedence over medical matters. A chapel was always found within the hospital or immediately attached to it. Spiritual care, however, was supplemented by generous portions of food and drink, administered by clerics with medical skills. Later both physicians and surgeons were hired to perform healing functions.[26]

The situation in Christian Spain contrasted with that found in Islamic hospitals. This hospital tradition, developed from sixth-century Byzantine models, led to the creation of *bimaristans*, homes of the sick, in the major urban centers of the Islamic empire. Secular institutions with a clear medical focus, these hospitals featured extensive staffs of physicians, surgeons, and apothecaries as well as well-stocked pharmacies and medicinal herb gardens. They engaged in both clinical and teaching activities and often acquired extensive libraries. This addition of an educational function to the hitherto religious and curative goals of the hospital influenced later developments in Christian Spain.[27]

Early in the sixteenth century, while medieval hospitals were declining all over Europe, Spain under the leadership of its Catholic Kings experienced a hospital boom, especially in cities conquered from the Moors. Granada (1511) and Valencia (1512), for example, each built large new hospitals. Hospital care, involving both soul and body, became an important tool for conversion and salvation. "Charity in the hospitals is extended to the Moor, to the Jew, to the heretic and gentile, and many are therein converted to the true faith of Jesus Christ, through the charity which is exercised therein toward them and others," wrote a chronicler of the Granada hospital.[28] Unaffected by the gradual secularization of hospitals elsewhere, and the transfer of poor relief to municipal authorities, Spanish hospitals continued during the sixteenth century to emphasize the religious significance of these institutions. The Spanish linkage of Catholicism and Crown gave rise to hospitals where both the spiritual and physical needs of the sick received attention.[29]

Medical Theory and Practice

Until the early sixteenth century, both medical theory and practice in Spain were based on the Galenic system of four humors as interpreted by medieval Islamic authors. For years the *Canon of Medicine*, written by Avicenna (980–1037), was the most popular text used in Spanish universities. In the 1530s, however, Spanish physicians trained in Italy brought the new humanism back to the Iberian peninsula; this Renaissance movement stressed a return to the wisdom of classical antiquity, in medicine the writings of Galen and Hippocrates, now available in their original Greek. Thanks to the appointment of some humanist physicians to chairs of *prima* and *vísperas*, the universities of Alcalá and Valencia became centers for the diffusion of this restored medical knowledge.[30]

Among the most prominent representatives of the reform movement was Andres Laguna (1510–1559), a prolific author and traveler, who published several Galenic works in Latin as well as numerous translations and commentaries from the Hippocratic corpus.[31] But the most famous Spanish writer of the century was probably Francisco Valles (1524–1592), professor of medicine at Alcalá from 1557 until 1572 and then personal physician and *protomédico general* under Philip II. Like Laguna and the other humanistic reformers, Valles preached a return to Hippocratic methods and traditions, stressing the importance of careful clinical observations and expressing scepticism toward previously used sources, especially the often erroneous and incomplete Latin translations from works in Arabic.

Toward the end of the century Luis Mercado (*ca.* 1525–1611), a graduate from the University of Valladolid, *protomédico*, and royal physician to Philip II, attempted to synthesize much of the medical knowledge acquired earlier, publishing his *Opera Omnia* (1594–1613) in four volumes. This work, reflecting the rising scholasticism of the Spanish Counter Reformation, attempted to assimilate all new insights into the prevailing Galenic system. Mercado's publications included a number of monographs on methodology, anatomy, physiology, hygiene, and such clinicopathological subjects as fevers, syphilis, and hereditary diseases.[32]

Because of links between the Crown of Aragon and leading Italian universities, human dissections were, after 1340, performed at the University of Montpellier in southern France, and the practice gradually spread south to Lérida (1391), Barcelona (1402), and Valencia (1477). Spurred by strong humanistic currents, the University of Valencia enthusiastically embraced the work of Andreas Vesalius (1514–1564), a pioneer in the study of human anatomy. Pedro Jimeno (*ca.* 1515–*ca.* 1558), a native of Valencia who had attended Vesalius' lectures at Padua between 1540–1543, led the movement to convert his university into one of the first institutions in all of Europe to teach Vesalian anatomy. The new instruction, based on systematic human dissections and Vesalius' *Fabrica* (1543), was continued at Valencia by Luis Collado (*ca.* 1520–1589), after Jimeno moved to Alcalá; a disciple of Collado's, Cosme de Medicina, carried the Vesalian tradition to Salamanca in 1551. The professor of anatomy at Valladolid, Juan Valverde de Hamusco (*ca.* 1520–*ca.* 1588), published in 1556 a textbook in Spanish based on the new anatomy.

One of the most important consequences of the Vesalian approach to human anatomy in Spain was the popularization of human dissections and description of normal and pathological findings. Francisco Valles of Alcalá was among the first to use data obtained at the autopsy table to buttress and expand theoretical arguments. With the help of the Valencian anatomist Pedro Jimeno, who carried out the dissections, Valles not only lectured on pathology in the autopsy room, but also incorporated his findings in a series of books designed to illustrate Galen's ideas on disease localization.[33]

Juan T. Porcell (1528–*ca.* 1580) of Sardinia further developed Valles' methods. A Salamanca graduate, Porcell found himself caring for about 800 inmates of the Nuestra Señora de Gracia Hospital in Zaragoza during the plague epidemic of 1564. Fearless of contagion, he systematically dissected fifty victims of the disease who had died in the hospital between May and December of that year, keeping careful records of their clinical course and the lesions observed at the autopsy. Porcell's monograph *Información y Curación de la Peste* (1565) employed simple statistical arguments and used postmortem findings to improve the classification of clinical forms of plague. Following Porcell, the employment of autopsies to ascertain possible causes of death and the seat of disease, especially during epidemics, became frequent in Spain and also in the colonies.[34]

During the early sixteenth century Spanish surgery continued to follow the late medieval works of the French surgeon Guy de Chauliac, which were translated into the vernacular languages of Spain and commented on by numerous authors. With the advent of humanism and the new Vesalian anatomy, however, a new generation of surgeons emerged from the Spanish universities and made significant contributions to contemporary surgical literature. This development, together with the inclusion of surgery in the medical curriculum and the new regulations issued by the *protomedicato*, allowed surgery to achieve a social and professional status in Renaissance Spain perhaps unequaled in Europe at that time. Spanish apprentices had at their disposal a series of excellent surgical treatises written on the basis of rich clinical experience and sound anatomical knowledge derived from systematic human dissections.[35]

Therapy was based on the Galenic model, which prescribed for most diseases a strategy of humoral removal, both as a prophylactic and therapeutic measure. Bloodletting, vomiting, purging, and sweating were routine treatments; herbal remedies, the most commonly used agents. The rationale for such procedures was that the removal of corrupt humors contributed to recovery by aiding the healing power of the human body.

With the recovery of classical texts in the sixteenth century, physicians such as Andres Laguna wrote new commentaries on Dioscorides, the Roman authority on medicinal plants. Laguna, who published in the vernacular, persuaded Philip II to follow the Italian example and establish botanical gardens in Spain for investigative purposes.[36] After midcentury, however, interest in medicinal plants from the New World quickly displaced the classical flora. Among the most prominent authors of the new materia medica were Nicolás Monardes (1507–1588) and Christóbal de

Acosta (*ca.* 1530–1580). The former, a graduate from Alcalá, cultivated the newly arriving plants in his botanical garden at Seville. Between 1565 and 1574 he published his *Historia Medicinal* in three parts, describing all drugs from America in terms of the four Galenic qualities of dryness, wetness, heat, and cold. He especially popularized the use of guaiacum and sarsaparilla.[37]

In the early 1500s guaiacum, the so-called holy wood from the New World, became a favorite remedy for the treatment of syphilis. Acting mainly as a diaphoretic, the decoction from the wood was believed to purify the blood by drawing off the poisons responsible for the venereal disease. Later in the century, however, physicians returned to using mercury in the treatment of syphilis as unfavorable clinical reports with guaiacum mounted.[38]

Spain boasted an alchemical laboratory erected under the sponsorship of Philip II and located at the royal palace of the Escorial. Workers there distilled a number of extracts from herbs, spices, and minerals to be used in the preparation of medicines and perfumes, an activity described in Francisco Valles' *Tratado de las Aguas Destiladas* (1592). Although the Swiss physician Paracelsus, an outspoken advocate of chemical remedies, had personally traveled through Spain between 1517 and 1519, his social position and personality precluded contacts with the country's medical elite. Nevertheless, Paracelsian ideas gradually diffused into Spanish medicine toward the end of the sixteenth century, leading briefly in 1591 to the establishment of a chair in chemical remedies at the University of Valencia.[39]

In all, Spanish medicine flourished during the Renaissance, especially between 1530 and 1580, when the physicians of Spain vigorously promoted a return to the classical authors and shifted their attention from scholastic concerns to clinical observations at the bedside, battlefield, and autopsy table. But the flowering of Spanish medicine did not last long. Intellectually and numerically depleted by the exodus of Jews and Moriscos, and stunted toward the end of the sixteenth century by a reversion to scholasticism under the influence of the Counter Reformation, medicine in Spain declined, never again to play so prominent a role in the development of medical theories, practices, and institutions.

MEDICINE IN NEW SPAIN

The region of central and southern Mexico called New Spain had achieved a notable degree of social and cultural development prior to the Spanish conquest of 1519–21. A number of warring native states had long vied for power and domination, imposing on their defeated neighbors heavy tributes in manpower and goods. At the time of the Spanish conquest the Triple Alliance of the Mexica, Tepaneca, and Acolhuaque controlled most of the territory, forming what is commonly designated as the Aztec empire. The supreme military and religious leader was Montezuma II.[40]

The size and health of the native population at the time of the conquest have been the subjects of much historical debate.[41] Recent research, however, has demonstrated the existence of a densely populated area in the central valley of Mexico, having a population of about three million, nearly half of whom lived in urban areas. The Aztec capital of Tenochtitlan, with about 150,000 to 200,000 inhabitants, surpassed all contemporary European cities in size.[42] The total population of the empire has been conservatively estimated at between five and ten million.

Despite intensive farming and use of the *chinampa* system of agriculture—floating plots of land distributed over the shallow lakes of central Mexico—the population seems to have lacked an adequate food supply.[43] Deforestation and soil erosion had already created badlands unfit for agriculture, while the absence of domesticated animals severely limited meat provisions. Sporadic starvation among the inhabitants of the valley seems to have already occurred by the middle of the fourteenth century. Food shortages and famines after crop failures recurred periodically, in four-year cycles, during the waning decades of the Aztec empire.[44]

Several authors have portrayed pre-Columbian Mexico as a virtually disease-free El Dorado, suddenly plunged into a chaos by frequent epidemics imported by the European conquerors.[45] This notion is based on the assumption that early inhabitants of the continent, trickling across the Bering Strait from Asia millennia ago, encountered a "cold screen" that drastically eliminated many pathogens and their vectors. Numerous so-called crowd diseases, requiring large numbers of susceptible subjects to maintain their viability (e.g., smallpox and measles), and other diseases with tropically based vectors, such as malaria and yellow fever, are be-

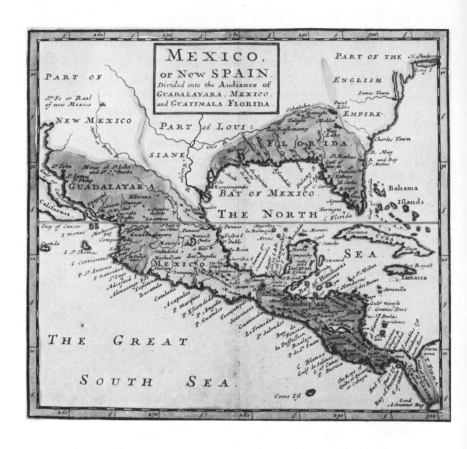

A map of Mexico, or New Spain. From Hermann Moll, *Atlas Manuale; or, A New Sett of Maps of All Parts of the Earth* . . . (London: Printed for J. Churchil and T. Childe, 1713). Courtesy of the State Historical Society of Wisconsin.

lieved to have been absent from the Americas until European colonization.[46]

Indeed both native morbidity and mortality from certain diseases introduced by the conquerors and new settlers suggest virgin soil epidemics reflecting a total lack of immunity to these ailments.[47] To compound the biological problem, socio-economical disruptions associated with the conquest and ensuing exploitation of the Indians created widespread famines and malnutrition in the already vulnerable population. Thus synergism between infection and malnutrition possibly contributed to stifling the necessary immunological responses, thereby accentuating the harmful impact of European diseases.[48]

The first epidemic severely to afflict the native population and undermine the Aztec empire occurred in 1520–21. Called *hueyzahuatl* in Nahuatl language and confidently identified as smallpox by contemporary Spanish chroniclers, the scourge was apparently carried to the coast near Veracruz by a black slave serving the conquistadors; and it spread rapidly inland, decimating the Indian population defending Tenochtitlan.[49] Ten years later, in 1531–32, a less malignant epidemic of smallpox, possibly combined with measles, followed, diffusing across the entire conquered territory. Then, between 1545 and 1548, New Spain suffered from a severe but as yet undiagnosed pestilence—*cocoliztli* in Nahuatl—having extremely high mortality. This disease is said to have killed a third of the remaining inhabitants of New Spain and caused widespread depopulation. Subsequent epidemics of smallpox, measles, and mumps continued to take a high toll in human lives, especially among native children in the highlands, who had no immunity, while the lowlands became virtually uninhabitable after the introduction of malaria, presumably through slaves brought over from Africa.[50] Another major epidemic of *cocoliztli* similar to the 1545 outbreak devastated the colony in 1576, spreading from Yucatán in the east to Chichimecas in the west and killing an estimated 300,000 to 400,000 people. After its first onslaught, the disease lingered in several regions until 1581.[51]

During the last two decades of the sixteenth century, colonial chroniclers reported periodic epidemics of measles and mumps among children, a sign of growing adult immunity. They also noted bouts of erysipelas, *tabardillo* (typhus and possibly typhoid fever), influenza, and diarrheal diseases clearly linked to malnutrition and

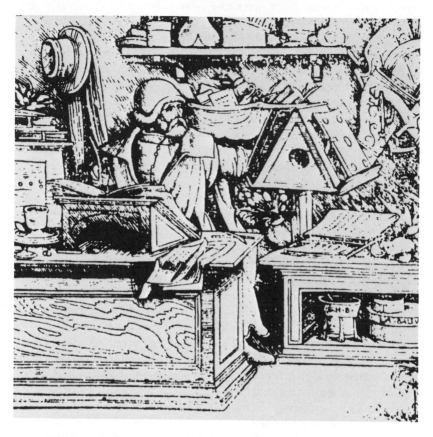

Woodcut depicting a sixteenth-century Spanish physician writing down his observations on the complexion and effects of green fruit. From Luis Lobera de Avila, *Vanquete de Nobles cavalleros e Modo de Bivir* (Augsburg: Henricus Stainerus, 1530), reproduced on p. 13 of *Catalogo del Fondo V. Peset Lllorca,* ed. by Juan A. Mico Navarro and Carolina Roig Castello, University of Valencia, 1983.

agricultural failures. The sustained demographic and economic impact of these diseases severely strained colonial institutions and commerce.[52]

Venereal disease, especially *bubas* or syphilis, assumed significant proportions among both Spanish settlers and natives. Although apparently pre-Columbian in origin,[53] venereal infections only emerged as an American health problem following European exploration and conquest, no doubt facilitated by the ensuing socio-economic breakdown and miscegenation.[54] Thus, barely a hundred years after the conquest, the native population of New Spain had sharply declined from an estimated five to ten million people to only one million, the compounded effect of warfare, epidemics, malnutrition, overwork, and the stresses of exploitation and acculturation.

Following the collapse of the Aztec empire in 1520, Cortés and other conquistadors expressed their admiration for native Mexican healers and their cures.[55] Although these men made no effort to conceal their preference for the resourceful Aztecs, other Spaniards found their magico-religious cosmology incompatible with Christian beliefs and European rationality. Thus, after 1525, a small number of Spanish physicians and surgeons began arriving in the rebuilt capital of the new colony.

Protomedicato

The regulation of medical practice in New Spain followed closely along lines established in the mother country. In 1525, shortly after the conquest of the Aztec empire, the municipal council of Mexico City appointed a barber-surgeon, Francisco de Soto, to act as *protomédico*, concerning himself with the regulation of medical practice and the precarious health of the city's inhabitants. In 1527 the licentiate Pedro López assumed that position, and from then on a succession of *protomédicos* demanded that all practitioners "explain by what right they practiced."[56] As in Spain, the reasons for this insistence are not hard to find. A number of irregular healers, both locals and foreigners, streamed into Mexico City, killing, in the eyes of the municipal council or *cabildo*, more people than they cured. To make matters worse, the first viceroy of New Spain received in 1535 royal instructions to require *limpieza de sangre* or purity of blood. Henceforth, no one of Moorish or Jewish descent could officially practice medicine or enter the universities of the New World. Native Aztec healers were equally unacceptable. This action significantly reduced the pool of health professionals eligible for certification by the *protomedicato*.[57]

The shortage of university-trained physicians and surgeons, a problem of considerable magnitude in Spain, was accentuated in New Spain. Contemporary testimony, for example, indicated that in 1545 there were apparently only four certified physicians in the entire capital. One of them, Juan de Alcázar, from Lérida, was preparing to return to Castile, seemingly overworked and in poor health. Another, Cristóbal Méndez, was in jail after arraignment by the Inquisition on suspicion of sorcery. That left only the licentiate Pedro López and the newly arrived Pedro de la Torre, an enterprising and opportunistic individual without a valid medical diploma and in legal difficulties with the *cabildo* of Veracruz, to serve the city. Both López and Alcázar were said to be "rich and prosperous."[58]

How wealthy these few physicians became is difficult to estimate, although descriptions of their "sumptuous" houses and "delightful" gardens are coupled with references to large households with slaves. Although the *cabildo* established a fee bill for physicians in 1535, the practitioners apparently ignored it, especially during epidemics. Ten years later, one citizen, Baltasar de Castro, protested that a physician's fee for an out-of-town house call was 6,000 *maravedís,* nearly the monthly salary of a professor of medicine in Spain.

Complaints about high fees, as well as the price and quality of drugs, were common in the early colony. Reports of unexamined apothecaries and exorbitant charges by barbers for bloodletting reached officials with great frequency. In response, municipal authorities moved cautiously, hoping to strengthen regulations without discouraging practitioners from settling in the colony. In 1540, for example, the *cabildo* allowed *protomédicos* to examine and certify midwives. Eight years later they approved a ceiling on fees for bloodletting, stipulating that Indians and black slaves should pay only half of the customary amount.[59] It is probable that these efforts at regulation, however laudable, fell victim to the laws of supply and demand. They may also have encouraged bribes and corruption.

In theory, at least, the power of the *protomédico* seemed awesome. From the beginning, however, his powers were constantly undermined by ever vigilant local and royal authorities who repeatedly took it upon themselves to carry out multiple "inspections" and "certifications."[60] The royal edict of 1570 appointing Francisco Hernández (1517–1587) as a special *protomédico* for New Spain, with powers to study all plants of medicinal value in the colony, limited his jurisdiction to roughly fifteen miles from his place of residence. All his decisions regarding medical examinations and licenses were subject to approval by the *royal audiencia*, the viceroy's governing body, or representatives of the Council of Indies in Spain. The senior judge of the *audiencia* was also empowered to follow Hernández during inspections and to sit with him during judicial proceedings.

When Hernández tried to function as a *protomédico* after his 1571 arrival in New Spain, he quickly learned that the *audiencia* intended to continue issuing licenses and titles and accepting appeals from persons convicted of practicing illegally. Despite his complaints to the crown and a special decree issued by Philip II in 1574, pressuring the viceroy to allow Hernández to carry out his functions, these conditions persisted during Hernández' entire stay in New Spain. As a result, the famous court physician apparently gave up his fruitless struggle and turned his attention completely to the scientific aspects of his mission.[61]

As Hernández discovered, because of the extreme shortage of health professionals in the colony, local viceroyal authorities time and again showed leniency in matters of certification and licensure, for example, tolerating practitioners who failed to prove purity of blood. The experience of Pedro de la Torre, previously identified as one of the few physicians residing in Mexico City in the 1540s, further illustrates the reluctance of authorities to enforce regulations strictly.[62]

After his arrival from Spain, a resident of Veracruz accused Torre of practicing medicine for pay without a valid license. When the matter came to the attention of the local magistrate, the physician contended that he had left his medical diploma in Spain, apparently a common excuse and plausible first line of defense. A few days later, however, he startled the authorities by presenting them with the required document. Unfortunately, it was obvious that the good doctor had simply erased the name of a recently deceased well-known practitioner and substituted his own. If

Torre assumed that the *cabildo* would be satisfied with the mere formality of a medical diploma, he miscalculated; the *cabildo* sent him to jail briefly before releasing him. Veracruz authorities urged Torre to send for his diploma in Spain, allowing him in the meantime to continue practicing medicine.

Unfortunately for Torre, his case was not forgotten, and when no diploma arrived from Spain, legal action was transferred from Veracruz to the *audiencia* in Mexico City. A verdict in 1545 found Torre guilty of violating the laws of the *protomedicato*, fined him an amount equivalent to half his property, and exiled him forever from New Spain. In his appeal, however, Torre enlisted an impressive array of colonists, including the bishop Juan de Zumarraga, to intercede in his behalf. Among the most weighty arguments in his favor was the fact that he had not neglected the treatment of black and Indian slaves during a recent epidemic, an expression of humanity or clever opportunism that set him apart from licensed colleagues busy treating the Spanish elite. Grateful slave owners provided another source of witnesses for the defense. Such was the need for medical manpower that the municipal powers of Mexico City appealed to the mercy of the *audiencia*, proposing that Torre be allowed to practice in the city if he successfully passed an examination to be given by established practitioners. Although the viceroy temporarily forced Torre to return to Spain, the resourceful doctor apparently forged a diploma from the University of Padua. With royal permission, Pedro de la Torre returned in 1547 to New Spain, where he successfully practiced in Veracruz, Mexico City, and Puebla.[63]

The last decades of the sixteenth century witnessed the arrival in New Spain of a few more university-trained physicians and surgeons and a number of Romance surgeons. Yet the system of inspections continued unabated, perhaps in part because it provided a welcome source of payoffs for participating functionaries. In response to developments in Spain, the authority of the *protomedicato* was strengthened after 1646 in that only qualified applicants with university degrees were allowed to practice legally, especially outside the larger urban areas; this prompted the development of an extensive illicit practice of medicine by empirics and *curanderos*, especially in rural areas.[64]

Among those in New Spain who filled the vacuum created by

the small number of physicians and surgeons were clerics, especially those belonging to the mendicant orders that labored in hospices and hospitals. Mine operators often took care of their Indian work force, and a large number of native healers, relying on the predominantly magico-religious Aztec medicine, ministered to Indians, blacks, and mestizos. Such *curanderismo* or folk healing, officially ridiculed by the Spaniards and later persecuted by the Inquisition, assumed an importance beyond furnishing health care to the vast majority of rural poor. In fact, by preserving religious and social values, the *curandero* became an essential figure in the survival of the traditional native culture. Use of magical procedures in healing helped native populations to maintain their identity and distinctiveness. Thus *curanderismo* became the most effective defense mechanism against Spanish acculturation, especially after 1620.[65]

Medical education

In 1570 Philip II justified the mission of Francisco Hernández to the New World by declaring: "Wishing that our subjects should enjoy a long life and preserve perfect health, we take care in providing them with physicians and teachers who will direct, teach, and cure their illnesses. With this goal in mind, we have established chairs of medicine and philosophy at the most important universities of the Indies."[66] The Royal and Pontifical University of Mexico had already been founded in 1551 by order of Charles V.[67] A quarter of a century later, in 1575, the Rector of the University, Gerónimo de Valdés Cárcamo, proposed the establishment of a medical chair. His recommendation, however, was rejected. Voting against it were three prominent physicians residing in the capital: Pedro López, Bartolomé de Valpuerta, and Florencio de Bique.

After assurances of funding from the king, however, the Mexican *audiencia* finally created a *prima* chair of medicine in 1578, following the regulations and curriculum then in use at the University of Salamanca. The first incumbent for a traditional four year term was Juan de la Fuente (*ca.* 1530–1595), a native of Palma de Mallorca. He had studied at the University of Siguenza and later taught at Seville before coming in 1563 to the colony, where he played an important role in the medical life of Mexico City. He delivered his first lecture, inaugurating formal medical education in New Spain, on January 7, 1579.[68]

After the establishment of the University of Mexico in 1551 and before the creation of medical chairs, physicians arriving in the colony with Spanish degrees needed to validate their diplomas and credentials according to *protomedicato* regulations in order to practice legally. The first to do so, in 1553, was Juan de Alcázar, a graduate from the University of Lérida, who had previously inspected the city's drugstores for the *cabildo*. De la Fuente, holder of the first medical chair, and Francisco Bravo, author of the earliest Mexican medical book, received new medical degrees from the University of Mexico in 1567 and 1570, respectively, on the basis of similar titles earned in Spain.

New degrees were awarded in a solemn formal ceremony held in a church. When Agustín Farfán received his Mexican doctorate in 1567, Viceroy Gastón de Peralta, Archbishop Alonso de Montúfar, and members of the royal *audiencia* all attended, as did university officials and faculty. Accompanied by his sponsor, Pedro López, Farfán demonstrated his eloquence and debating skills against the rector and two well-known physicians, discussing a question about the role of blood in disease. Following the highly stylized debate and several speeches, Farfán received his new doctoral insignias, ring, spurs, sword, and velvet hat.[69]

The creation of the *prima* chair of medicine in 1578 led to the admission of the first medical students in New Spain. As in Spain, all candidates had to possess a bachelor of arts degree and to demonstrate purity of blood and adherence to Catholic dogma. To obtain the bachelor of medicine degree, students studied for four years. During the first two, they read a number of Hippocratic works dealing with humoral theory, temperaments, the nature of man, fevers, and pulse. In the third year, students listened to the aphorisms of Hippocrates and the *Ad Almansorem* of Rhazes; in the fourth, they studied Galen's *Metodo Medendi*.[70]

For the first twenty years these subjects were all taught by one professor who lectured daily from ten to eleven o'clock in the morning. Since appointment to the *prima* chair lasted only four years, Juan de la Fuente applied for additional terms in 1582, 1586, 1590, and 1594, and, being the only candidate, he was reappointed each time. The first three graduates, all licenciates, received their diplomas in 1584, six years after classes had begun and two years after receiving their bachelor of medicine degrees. By the end of the sixteenth century, approximately nineteen baccalaureate and twelve doctoral degrees of medicine had been awarded. The university offered no training for Latin surgeons.[71]

A second chair of medicine, *vísperas,* was not created at the University of Mexico until 1598. After the usual *oposición* or academic competition, the authorities elected Juan de Plascencia, an alumnus who had received his degree in 1593. Plascencia lectured from three to four o'clock in the afternoon, during which he read various classics on pathology and disease. His chair was considered temporary because it had no permanent funding; in 1626 it carried a salary of only 300 pesos. Mexican salaries were, by Spanish standards, quite low. The professor of *prima* received 500 pesos, compared with 700 pesos given to the professors of theology and law. Secretarial help at the university received 200 pesos per year.[72]

In 1621, the University of Mexico received a proposal from Cristóbal Hidalgo y Vendaval to establish a third chair, of *Metodo Medendi* or therapeutic methodology. In his request, Hidalgo, a Creole physician who had obtained his doctorate from the university in 1607, stressed the importance of the subject and offered to teach without compensation. Since his petition involved no financial obligation, it won quick approval from the authorities, and Hidalgo assumed his chair a month after submitting his proposal. His lectures were scheduled between four and five o'clock in the afternoon, following those given by the teacher of *vísperas.*[73] Hidalgo's selection of Galen's *Metodo Medendi* as a text for his course suggests that he had no interest in discussing the fusion of Spanish and Aztec therapies. He stressed the medical classics and left up to the initiative of his students the connecting of the medical theory of these books with the realities of colonial practice.

That same year the university also founded a chair of anatomy and surgery, responding to a decree issued in 1617 by Philip III, who wanted to improve medical education both at home and in the colonies. In the future, no Spanish or Spanish American university could award a bachelor of medicine degree unless its students had taken courses in *prima, vísperas,* and anatomy-surgery. To enforce this requirement, the *protomedicato* was enjoined from examining medical graduates who could not prove attendance at such courses.

Although an early medical alumnus, Rodrigo Muñoz, offered to teach anatomy and surgery without pay, the faculty eventually selected Cristóbal Hidalgo y Vendaval for the post. In justifying their appointment, officials claimed that Hidalgo had acquired extensive surgical experience in convents, hospitals, and monasteries. Moreover, his present academic duties already included some surgical therapeutics. Hidalgo accepted the new post without stipend or salary. Apparently he only lectured to students because compulsory anatomical dissections were not required until 1645. The University of Mexico, by fulfilling Philip III's royal decree, acquired a full complement of medical chairs to train its students. The institutional transfer of medical education to New Spain was complete.[74]

It is significant that almost three decades passed between the foundation of the university and the creation of a medical chair. At the very least it suggests that colonial authorities did not consider such studies to be an effective remedy for the chronic shortage of physicians and the proliferation of irregular healers and quacks. The relatively small number of physicians trained by the university during its early years indicates that the authorities were wise to look elsewhere for a solution of their problem.

Given the constant trickle of Spanish graduates arriving in the colony to treat the Spanish urban elite, the university probably saw little reason to endow a new chair in medicine. Academic rivalries and the primacy of theology probably also hampered efforts to expand the faculty. Not surprisingly, the medical profession in the capital seems to have been equally reluctant to support formal medical training; at least there is no indication that any of its members pressured the academic authorities into creating a chair. Because of the shortage of competent healers, these physicians were in great demand and were able to exact high fees for their services; they had little interest in fostering more competition. The opposition of Pedro López, Bartolomé de Valpuerta, and Florencio de Bique to the creation of the first medical chair certainly suggests such a motive. More important, the delay also reflects the low esteem that sixteenth-century colonial authorities accorded to medicine as an effective instrument in curbing epidemics and restoring health. The devastating epidemics that desolated New Spain in 1576–77 seem to have given little, if any, impetus to the creation of medical professorships.

Medical education in both Spain and the colonies stressed a rational orientation to matters of health and disease that appealed primarily to *gente de razón*—people of reason. For the vast majority of New Spain's residents, whether Indian, black, or mestizo, sickness continued to have a supernatural significance that no logical exposition of humors, temperaments, and qualities could fully explain or justify. For these people, eloquence and debating skills, philosophical argumentations and flawless quotations of texts sharpened through numerous examinations and *oposiciones*, meant little. Hippocrates had indeed come to the colonies, but he was known only among the educated elite.

Hospitals

Hospitals in New Spain also followed Spanish models. As early as 1502, Isabel of Castile instructed Nicolás de Ovando, Columbus' successor as governor of the island of Hispaniola, "to build hospitals where the poor can be housed and cured, whether Christians or Indians."[75] The royal order instituted a social welfare system called *beneficencia* developed by the Spanish rulers and the Church to insure the wellbeing of colonial inhabitants and to facilitate evangelization of the indigenous population.[76] Epidemics and war had left millions homeless, hungry, and sick, needing food and shelter, hope and care. As Pedro de Gante, a Franciscan friar, confided in a letter to Charles V in 1532, medical care could be employed in New Spain as a tool to convert Indians to Christianity, just as the Castilian rulers had used it to convert the Moors.[77]

Indeed the mendicant orders engaged in the spiritual conquest of the new territories played an active role in founding hospitals. The Franciscans arrived in New Spain in 1523 and scattered throughout the colony. The Dominicans followed them three years later, settling especially in Oaxaca and Morelos. In 1533 the Augustinians entered the regions of Michoacán, Guerrero, and Hidalgo. Toward the end of the century the *cofradía* or brotherhood of St. Hippolytus, a hospital association begun in the City of Mexico and the first aboriginal congregation to receive official papal approval, also began filtering into the countryside. And in

1602, Viceroy Mendoza Luna allowed the Brotherhood of St. John of God to enter New Spain and begin their charitable hospital work.[78]

Support for the establishment of hospitals came from both private and public sectors. Because the state allowed private parties to found charitable institutions, a number of hospitals in New Spain owed their existence to the generosity of individual donors. Church-mediated gifts in the form of a *memoria* or rents obtained from property bequested to the Church in perpetuity also allowed private citizens to contribute to hospitals. Royal subsidies derived from Indian tribute, profits from monopolies and pharmacies, and portions of the tithe often went to that support. In this activity the Church and the Crown successfully worked together under the aegis of a peculiarly Spanish church-state relationship.[79]

There were two types of hospitals in New Spain: general and specialized. In cities, general hospitals, which took care of sick Spaniards and Indians of both sexes, were usually located near the central plaza and the church. No doubt prompted by the repeated epidemics and the conviction that miasma, or bad air, caused disease, a royal decree in 1573 required that "when a city, village or place be founded, the hospitals for the non-contagious sick are to be placed next to the church, and for the contagious sick, errected in an elevated place where no ill winds passing through the hospitals are going to hurt the population."[80]

In 1521 the conquistador Hernando Cortés founded the first general hospital in New Spain, in the City of Mexico. Named Hospital de la Concepción de Nuestra Señora, this institution was designed specifically to care for the sick poor, both Spaniards and Indians; however, it excluded patients suffering from leprosy, syphilis, madness, and St. Anthony's fire. Cortés financed the establishment from his own personal fortune as a gesture of thanksgiving and penance, and he made elaborate arrangements in his will for a permanent endowment. The first physicians arriving in the city from Spain, Pedro López and Cristóbal de Ojeda, and the barber-surgeon Francisco de Soto practiced in this hospital.[81]

Other early hospitals were founded in Veracruz, the unhealthful point of disembarkation for those coming into the colony, and throughout Michoacán, the region west of the capital and the center of Franciscan missionary activity. By 1600, there were twelve hospitals in the area surrounding the City of Mexico; Michoacán had approximately seventy-two, Colima in the west had nine. Archbishop Alonso de Mantúfar, a Dominican, declared in 1554 that the establishment of hospitals was the most important development in the life of the new colony.[82]

Special hospitals existed for patients believed to be suffering from leprosy. Traditionally dedicated in Europe to Saint Lazarus, these establishments or lazarettos were generally located outside of towns to insure the isolation of their inmates. In the early 1520s, Cortés built the Hospital de San Lázaro in Tlaxpana, outside the City of Mexico. In 1539, Bishop Juan de Zumárraga founded the Hospital del Amor de Dios exclusively for patients suffering from syphilis, since they were excluded from Cortés' general hospital. In 1567 Bernardino Alvarez, an affluent former conquistador, erected the Hospital de San Hipólito on the outskirts of Mexico City and dedicated it to convalescents and mental patients.[83]

In 1555 the colonial authorities in Mexico City discussed in earnest the establishment of hospitals exclusively devoted to Indians, who composed about 80 percent of the city's inhabitants. If the natives could be congregated in one place during the epidemics, it would be easier for the clergy to administer last rites. Aided by new instructions from Philip II a year later, local authorities expanded and rebuilt the Hospital Real San José de los Naturales, originally established in the early 1530s by Fray Pedro de Gante, and the Franciscans, for the care of Indians. With eight wards, this establishment could accommodate more than 200 sick and destitute Indians.[84]

The reorganized hospital was supported by Indian tribute, the *medio real de hospital*. Each Indian village in New Spain was enjoined to pay the institution one Spanish bushel of corn out of every hundred collected. Additional income came from items willed by patients to the hospital. The new building, completed in 1556, housed one ward for contagious cases and another for persons suffering from rabies. An ambulatory department treated emergency cases. The staff consisted of five chaplains, two physicians, two surgeons, and various apprentices. As in certain Spanish hospitals of the period, autopsies of patients dying in the institutions were permitted in order to ascertain cause of death.[85]

Although the health care of natives in the City of Mexico and its environs remained in the hands of the Crown, elsewhere Franciscans and Augustinians ran hospitals exclusively for Indians. Most of these institutions were erected without specific donations and were maintained by the contributions of religious *cofradías*. The sick usually resided in a small building adjacent to the church or convent. The hospitals of Tiripetio (1537), Uruapán (1561), Taximaroa (1580), San Martín Turundero (1595), Cuitzeo (1550), Peribán (1541), and Tarecuato (1541) were all located in the province of Michoacán and surrounding regions, an area with a large concentration of Indians.

The Hospital de Santa Cruz, established in 1569 at Huaxtepec by Bernardino Alvarez, well known for his charitable works, merits special mention. This hospital was located about fifty miles from the City of Mexico, on a beautiful site previously used as a retreat by Aztec rulers. Many plants, including a large number of medicinals that had been collected as spoils of war from throughout the country, grew in Montezuma's gardens, a popular spa, which, according to the natives, possessed healing powers. Alvarez' establishment was designed to care for convalescents and patients suffering from chronic ailments, who were shuttled from Mexico's St. Hippolytus Hospital by members of the Brotherhood of Charity dedicated to this saint. The physicians at the Hospital de Santa Cruz used native herbs to treat a variety of medical problems, including syphilis.[86]

When the *protomédico* Francisco Hernández visited the hospital, perhaps in 1574, he learned a great deal about medicinal plants and returned to the capital with a rich harvest of information. Gregorio López (*ca.* 1542-*ca.* 1596), a hermit and medical author, had a similar experience during his stay as a patient. His unpublished "Tesoro de la Medicinas" contains observations concerning medical treatments with botanical remedies. The excellent reputation of the Hospital de Santa Cruz as a spa with innovative therapeutics attracted patients from all over New Spain and from as far away as Guatemala and Peru.[87]

Among the most distinctive of New Spain's private hospitals were the so-called pueblo-hospitals established by Vasco de Quiroga (1477–1565), a judge of the second Mexican *audiencia*. Like other Spanish officials and clerics in the colony, Quiroga desired to educate and convert the Indians as well as ameliorate the abuses they were suffering at the hands of their new lords. Influenced by Thomas More's *Utopia*, Quiroga advocated the creation of pueblos composed of 6,000 extended families, each consisting of ten to sixteen married couples from the same lineage. A central feature of each settlement was a hospital containing separate facilities for patients with contagious diseases. A *mayordomo* (superintendent) and a *dispensero* (literally a dispenser of first aid) administered the hospital, which was also served by a physician, surgeon, and apothecary.[88]

With permission from the Spanish Crown, Quiroga brought his utopian project to fruition in 1531 with the founding of the Hospital de Santa Fé de Mexico near the capital city. The core of this new settlement was a group of young, acculturated Indians who had grown up in the early Spanish monasteries. In 1534 Quiroga started a second pueblo, the Hospital de Santa Fé de la Laguna, near Lake Patzcuaro, in the province of Michoacán. Like the hospital at Sante Fé de Mexico, this one served as a refuge for poor, orphaned, or sick Indians who gravitated to the pueblo. Quiroga's work attracted widespread attention and royal support, leading to his appointment as bishop of the newly organized diocese of Michoacán in 1536—this in spite of his former nonreligious status. In 1580, seventeen years after Quiroga's death, the pueblo hospitals were still flourishing even though the total number of inhabitants was decreasing. At about this time Santa Fé de Mexico had a population of about 120 families while Santa Fé de la Laguna reported 100.[89]

As an experiment in converting and educating Indians, Quiroga's scheme proved successful. In providing health care, however, it seems to have been less efficacious, especially after the establishment of hospitals for natives in the City of Mexico and in the province of Michoacán. Evidence for this conclusion comes from a protracted legal battle waged in 1572 by the authorities in the capital to take over the richly endowed Santa Fé de Mexico. The state claimed that Quiroga's main objective, healing the sick, was being neglected in violation of his will. Testimony disclosed that the hospital had cared for only a handful of sick inhabitants and a few nonresidents in the preceding months. Although the Council of Indies eventually rejected the proposed annexation, it seems clear that depopulation following epidemics and competition with other urban developments presented serious obstacles to the growth of the pueblo-hospitals.[90]

By the early seventeenth century, New Spain possessed an impressive network of approximately 128 hospitals, strategically located in the most densely populated areas and along major roads. Writing in 1583, Bishop Pedro Moya de Contreras declared that "in all Indian villages with the rank of *cabeceras* or head towns, there are hospitals built with the labor, money, and alms of the Indians themselves."[91] In spite of chronic financial difficulties and occasional corruption, one of Spain's most impressive colonizing efforts in the New World had achieved its primary goal.

In many respects the hospitals of New Spain served a social function similar to those in the mother country. Even the effort to use them to convert the Indians had been anticipated in Spain, on a much smaller scale, when the Spanish kings employed hospitals to help Christianize the reconquered Moors. The novel feature of hospitals in New Spain was their role in reversing the dispersal of the indigenous population, frightened by ruthless *encomenderos* and threatened by disease. Hospitals attracted Indians not only temporarily, such as during epidemics, but permanently, for example in the pueblos.[92] With their large patient populations and *cofradías,* they functioned as centers for Spanish acculturation. Both religious celebrations and medical routines allowed the natives not only to learn Christian dogma and values, but a new language and a sense of community.

The hospitals affected public health both positively and negatively. Congregating the natives during epidemics no doubt spread contagion, especially since isolation procedures were then largely ineffective. Whether removing the sick to hospitals decreased the spread of disease among the remaining population remains unclear. Nevertheless, the comfort, rest, and nourishment given to those hospitalized probably saved many lives by improving their nutrition and resistance to disease. Above all, hospital care for the Indians bolstered morale in times of hunger and despair, abuse and pain.

The hospitals of New Spain occasionally fostered medical science by furnishing patient populations for clinical experimentation with native remedies. They also furthered the study of anatomy and pathology by allowing autopsies to be performed on deceased patients, and, more important, they counterbalanced the scholasticism of the universities by providing physicians with practical clinical experience.

Medical theory and practice

In his instructions to Francisco Hernández in 1570, Philip II not only stressed the potential benefits that would accrue from a knowledge of New World medicinal plants, but spelled out the methods to acquire the desired data. The king directed the *proto-médico* to gather information "from all physicians, surgeons, Spanish and Indian herbalists, and other curious persons with such abilities who evidently could understand and know something, and obtain in general an account of all medicinal herbs, trees, plants, and seeds that exist in a given province." Furthermore, he ordered Hernández to ask informants about the faculties, temperaments, and dosages of these medicines and, if possible, to perform clinical tests or at least secure affidavits from experts certifying all therapeutic claims.[93]

These royal instructions reflected the great interest of both the Crown and Spanish medical circles in American drugs. Their concern was more than scientific; it stemmed as well from economic considerations related to trade in spices and drugs, an issue of paramount importance. As mentioned earlier, guaiacum, the holy wood from the Caribbean islands, was already being employed in Spain by 1516 to treat syphilis, and its use spread rapidly to other European countries. The profits made by those who imported this wood from the New World suggested that fortunes awaited the discovery of new remedies.[94]

Since the time of Columbus, accounts of miraculous cures with New World plants had flooded Spain. In a letter to Charles V, written in 1521, the conquistador Hernando Cortés vividly described the herb sellers of Tlatelolco and their numerous medicines.[95] Three decades later, the Crown received a manuscript titled "Libellus de Medicinalibus Indorum Herbis" from the Franciscan Colegio de Santa Cruz in Tlatelolco, an institution devoted to the education of young Indians and to the preservation of Aztec culture. This document, a Latin translation of an Aztec work written by a native healer, Martín de la Cruz, summarized traditional medical knowledge. It also included hundreds of drawings depicting a great variety of medicinal plants. Although it was never published, this work proved to the royal court that herbal riches awaited the colonists.[96]

Hernández closely followed the methodology suggested by

Philip II for gathering medical information. As revealed in his letters and reports, he viewed Aztec medicine within the context of his own humoral pathology and therapeutics and constantly sought to explain favorable effects in those terms. He often tasted medicinal products in order to classify them and assign them fundamental Galenic qualities, a method that more than once made him gravely ill. Stripped of their magico-religious context, native practices made little sense to a foreign practitioner who adhered to a naturalistic system of medicine, and Hernández often expressed doubts about claims made by Indians if he could not readily find humoral explanations.

Hernández summarized his criticisms of Aztec medicine in a manuscript titled "De Antiquitatibus Novae Hispaniae," which discussed Indian customs, ceremonies, and laws.[97] Written during the early 1570s, Hernández' comments typify the reactions of learned Spanish physicians who had occasion to observe native healing. His foremost complaint was that Aztec healers or *ticitl* did not study the nature of individual diseases or differentiate between individual ailments. In his view, their histories and examinations of the sick were too superficial to facilitate differential diagnoses. He was also dismayed by what he felt were insufficient dietary recommendations for the sick, a fundamental part of his therapeutic regimen. The Indians, moreover, did not perform phlebotomies, so common in European practice, but restricted their bloodletting to occasional scarifications. Above all, Hernández thought that native remedies were prescribed irrationally and without enough flexibility to deal with changing clinical situations. Hence he concluded that Aztec healers were merely empirics, rigidly using their materia medica according to traditions passed on from generation to generation.[98]

Hernández believed that such practices stifled the natives' capacity to take full advantage of their abundant medicinal flora. In addition, he felt that ignorance of elementary pharmaceutical skills led to a dangerous use of many potentially valuable drugs, the poisonous qualities of which were unchecked by artful compounding.[99]

Hernández' reservations about indigenous medicine must be kept in mind when analyzing the early medical literature of New Spain, our best source of information about medical theory and practice in the colonies. All of those who wrote on this subject were Spanish physicians and surgeons motivated by a desire to correct the same deficiencies Hernández had perceived and thereby recast Aztec medicine according to classical Hippocratic and Galenic models. In their opinion, a theoretical knowledge of humors and qualities was needed in order to understand the nature of disease, to distinguish between clinical pictures, and to render a correct prognosis. Likewise, they thought that humoralism could transcend blind Aztec empiricism and enable the establishment of rational therapeutics, flexible enough to incorporate many valuable elements from the native pharmacopoeia.

The first medical work published in New Spain, a book titled *Opera Medicinalia* (1570), was written by the Spanish physician Francisco Bravo (*ca*. 1525–1595). Originally from Seville, Bravo received his M.D. from the University of Osuna and also studied at Alcalá de Henares before moving to the colonies in the late 1560s. Months before the appearance of his book, he received a new degree from the University of Mexico and decided to remain in the capital city to practice. Bravo played a prominent role in the professional medical affairs of the colony and was appointed *protomédico* in 1587, 1592, and 1593.[100]

Bravo's work, written in Latin, was an erudite treatise full of references to classical and Islamic authors. In four separate essays it successively examined a disease the Spanish called *tabardete* (probably a form of typhus or typhoid fever), venesection in pleuresy, the Hippocratic doctrine of critical days, and the nature and properties of sarsaparilla. The author's views, typical of the times, reflected the interests of a well-educated Renaissance physician writing for his peers. Both the essays on venesection and on critical days consisted of a series of logical arguments buttressed with quotations from classical and contemporary authorities. Only the discussions of *tabardete* and sarsaparilla incorporated Bravo's new colonial experience. His previous encounters in Seville with *tabardete* made him an acute observer of the clinical and epidemiological aspects of the malady. In the Hippocratic tradition, Bravo summarized the sanitary conditions prevalent at the time the disease appeared in the City of Mexico, noting the polluted lakes and the dangers of miasmatic exhalations trapped in the valley by surrounding mountains. *Tabardete* apparently affected inhabitants year round; it was both contagious and highly lethal.[101]

The final essay, on the sarsaparilla root, reflected the interest expressed in Europe about using this plant to treat fevers and syphilis. Bravo took pains to demonstrate that, contrary to the opinion derived from native healers, the root was hot and dry. His detailed morphological description of the plant was supplemented by two drawings, the first published images of New World botanicals. Bravo's *Opera Medicinalia* represents a high point in sixteenth-century medical literature and compares favorably with contemporary European publications on the subject. Yet its usefulness was greatly restricted because only a handful of colonial practitioners were able to read the volume.[102]

Bravo's scholarly treatise was followed in 1578 by a surgical treatise written in Spanish by Alonso López de Hinojosos (*ca.* 1534–1597) and titled *Suma y Recopilación de Cirugía.* The contrast between these two publications and their authors could not have been greater. López de Hinojosos was an apprentice-trained barber-surgeon and phlebotomist, who had practiced in Spain before immigrating to the colonies around 1567. Employed at both the Hospital Real de los Naturales and Cortés' Hospital de la Concepción de Nuestra Señora in the City of Mexico, López acquired extensive clinical experience and, as superintendent of the former institution, administrative skills. In spite of his marginal professional status, be built up an excellent reputation as a surgeon among both Spaniards and Indians. In 1576, with a deadly epidemic of *cocoliztle* (pestilence) raging in the city, he carried out a series of autopsies under the supervision of Francisco Hernández, in which he tried to determine the cause of this scourge and thus find an effective remedy for it. Well known for his piety and hospital donations, López joined the Jesuits in 1585, becoming *portero* or gate keeper at the Colegio Mayor de San Pedro y San Pablo in the capital city, where he continued to see patients until his death in 1597.[103]

The first edition of his *Suma y Recopilación de Cirugía,* based in large part on the medieval works of Guy de Chauliac, appeared in 1578. In his dedication to the archbishop of Mexico, López declared that "this little service is for poor people and especially the Indians like those under my care, so that their surgical ailments can be cured as they have been so far by myself." His book was written, he declared in the introduction, "for anyone who could read and lived outside the capital on *estancias,* in small towns

Sy M M A,

Y RECOPILACION

DE CHIRVGIA, CON VN
Arte para fagrar muy vtil y prouechofa.

COMPVESTA POR MAES-
tre Alonfo Lopez, natural de los Inojofos.
Chirujano y enfermero del Ofpital de
S. Iofeph de los Yndios, defta muy
infigne Ciudad de Mexico.

DIRIGIDO AL ILL. Y R.
S. Don P. Moya de Contreras, Arçobifpo
de Mexico y del côcejo de fu Mageft.

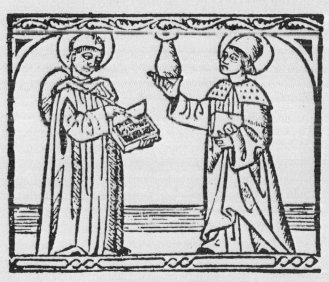

EN MEXICO,
Por Antonio Ricarco. 1578.

Title page of Alonso López de Hinojosos' surgical treatise, *Suma y Recopilación de Cirugía* (Mexico City, 1578).

near mines, and in remote areas lacking useful remedies."[104] He deplored the jargon of surgical texts, even those written for Romance surgeons, and thus wrote in simple language accessible to the irregular practitioners who provided the bulk of health care in the colony. He often recommended native herbs—over fifty in all—"born in this land through the mercy of God."

Of particular interest is López' description of the devastating epidemic of *cocoliztle* in 1576, which provides a glimpse of how civic leaders in Mexico City responded to this highly contagious and deadly disease. Viceroy Martín Enríquez convened a conference of prominent physicians to advise him. The Hospital Real de los Naturales, which had only about two hundred beds, took in as many patients as it could, leaving other ailing natives to subsist on donations of food and clothing distributed by secular and mendicant clerics. The archbishop ordered these men to comb the Indian quarter of the city, hearing confessions, dispensing sacraments, and, in López' words, "wanting more the salvation of the Indians' souls than their [bodily] health."[105]

Because so little was known about the disease, the viceroy ordered physicians to carry out autopsies of Indians who had died from it. Under the direction of the *protomédico,* Francisco Hernández, López de Hinojosos indeed dissected several corpses in early 1577. To Hernández, the pathological findings suggested poisoning, and therefore he recommended a neutralizing regimen based on the administration of theriac, a cure-all containing opiates, alcohol, and more than fifty other compounds. In addition to theriac, López prescribed the root of *coanenepilli,* a native antidote with antispasmodic and febrifuge properties.[106]

Another colonial work that incorporated Aztec therapeutics appeared first under the title *Tractado Brebe de Anathomia y Chirurgia* (1579) and later, in a revised edition, as *Tractado Brebe de Medicina* (1592). Its author, Agustín Farfán (1532–1604), was a Spanish physician from Seville who had studied medicine there and at Alcalá de Henares. Farfán left Spain in 1557 and ten years later obtained a new diploma from the University of Mexico. Temporarily appointed *protomédico* in 1568, Farfán joined the Augustinian order a year later and changed his name to Friar Agustín Farfán.[107] Farfán was one of the most distinguished physicians of New Spain during the last quarter of the sixteenth century.

He alternated his medical practice with extended inspection tours of convents throughout the colony, and it is possible that he cooperated with Francisco Hernández after 1574 in therapeutic experiments at the Hospital Real de los Naturales.

In the first chapter of his *Tractado Brebe de Medicina,* Farfán clearly identified his intended audience:

> Those who are physicians may wish to read my treatise because it is a brief compendium of what the greatest authorities have taught over a long time. However, I don't write for them but instead for those who live where there are no physicians. With divine help I shall try to be clear so that all can understand me. The remedies will be the most common ones to be found. . . . I trust that God will make the remedies wherever He will be.[108]

Time and again when writing about common ailments, Farfán recommended indigenous herbs, often as substitutes for scarce European drugs. He couched his suggestions in simple language, like that used in kitchen-medicine recipes. He assured his readers that he had tried the various remedies and found them useful. For example, in writing about remedies for menstrual irregularities, he noted that

> those I put down here have been of great use to me, they have never been unavailable, and can be made everywhere. As I have already said, what is good in this treatise is that the remedies can be made even when the sick do not have a drugstore [nearby]. I beg you to use them and you shall be cured with God's favor even if the ailments appear incurable.[109]

In all, Farfán recommended nearly sixty indigenous medicinals, including pulverized avocado pits as an antidiarrheic; the extract of agave leaves mixed with honey as an expectorant; chili peppers, vanilla, and rhubarb as purgatives; hot chocolate as a laxative; copal as an astringent resin; and sarsaparilla as a diaphoretic. He prescribed pits from sapota fruits for asthma, cramps, and headaches; Artemisia Mexicana, a herb, for leg swellings, for intestinal worms, and to promote menstruation; and corn, ingested in the form of hot tortillas or applied directly on painful areas of the abdomen, for colics. To treat syphilis, he advised using a decoction made from guaiacum.[110]

In a brief chapter on anatomy, addressed to surgeons who

must "cut, open, and cauterize," Farfán declared that a lack of anatomical knowledge caused surgeons to "make irremediable errors every day." Often quoting from Hippocrates, Galen, and Avicenna, he presented in a basic head-to-toe arrangement the body's major vessels, nerves, muscles, and internal organs. In a chapter on surgery, he frequently recommended salves made from native herbs.

The writings of Bravo, López, and Farfán testify to the emergence of a novel medical literature written for a people who lacked an adequate supply of learned physicians and thus depended mostly on irregular Spanish and native practitioners. Their texts were all written in Spanish and in straightforward language, and their recommendations were simple to follow. Their medical theories, however, continued to be based on classical models of physiology and pathology that ascribed changes to bodily humors and their qualities.

The incorporation of traditional Aztec remedies into colonial medical practice occurred because of their practical value and availability. This "reverse acculturation" took place in part because Spanish drugs were scarce, expensive, and often of poor quality. Moreover, potent native plants seemed to cure specific symptoms and could be prepared simply, without resorting to cumbersome Old World procedures designed to enhance pharmacological action. As colonial authors pointed out, such simples could even be prepared at home if no drugstore was nearby.[111]

But Aztec drugs could only be incorporated into the existing European materia medica on terms compatible with Greco-Roman humoralism. Colonial practitioners, observing certain clinical effects produced by native herbs, ascribed specific qualities to them. For example, because sarsaparilla caused considerable perspiration when ingested in various types of drinks, such as teas, Farfán declared, in the vocabulary of traditional theory, that the root possessed a second and third degree of hotness, and he therefore employed it in situations where excess humoral coldness was suspected. Such behavior suggests that Spanish physicians rarely used native drugs as dictated by local tradition and that new additions to the pharmacopoeia failed to challenge the basic tenets of medical theory and therapeutics prevailing in Europe. Most physicians continued to attribute symptoms and pathological changes to humoral disturbances and to rely on the depletion of harmful fluids—by bloodletting, purging, vomiting, and sweating—as the key strategy to restoring a normal balance.

CONCLUSION

During the first century of its existence, New Spain imported medical institutions, personnel, and knowledge from the mother country. Instead of trying to learn from Aztec medicine, the new Spanish settlers chose to suppress it, resorting to the same bureaucratic and religious constraints that had driven Islamic medicine underground in Spain. As a result there emerged a form of popular medical practice, called *curanderismo,* that not only served the majority of Indians, mestizos, and blacks, but preserved the remnants of native culture.

However, the *gachupines,* as the natives of Spain became known in America, generally found the magico-religious and empirical procedures of Aztec medicine to be unacceptable. They insisted on regulating medical practice in accordance with the laws of the *protomedicato,* but the extreme shortage of qualified health professionals forced them constantly to show leniency to persons practicing illegally. Although the universities of New Spain established chairs of medicine, they trained only a small number of physicians and closely followed Old World models.

The hospitals of New Spain also adhered to principles developed in Spain. In New Spain, however, they acquired greater importance since the Indians, threatened by European diseases and exploitative masters, needed a sanctuary capable of protecting them from extinction. Although the medical benefits of hospitalization were dubious at best, these institutions played a key role in religious conversion, Spanish acculturation, and social control.

Spanish physicians and surgeons also brought to the colonies the medical theories and practices common in Europe. On the basis of such theories, colonial practitioners adopted a considerable number of native plants for therapeutic purposes. In doing so, they were simply following their colleagues in Spain, who also employed medicines found in the New World. In New Spain, however, such factors as availability, cost, and simplicity of prepara-

52	GUENTER B. RISSE

tion probably increased the use of these products. But in spite of the adoption of native remedies, the medical system brought over from Europe remained intact.

By the early decades of the seventeenth century, the transfer of institutions and personnel to New Spain was virtually complete. The *protomedicato* continued to regulate medical practice until Mexico became independent in the early nineteenth century. No new hospitals appeared for almost 200 years, and the surviving institutions maintained a precarious existence, constantly threatened by shortages of funds. Finally, because of the intellectual isolation imposed by Spain on its colonies during the Counter Reformation, medical theory and practice in New Spain stagnated.

NOTES

I am indebted to Drs. José M. López Piñero (University of Valencia), Francisco Guerra (Universidad de Alcalá de Henares), and Juan Somolinos Palencia (Mexican Society for the History and Philosophy of Medicine) for providing me with the necessary articles and books to write this work.

1. There is no recent summary of Spanish medicine in English. The most complete list of personalities, events, and dates can be found in an editorial by Fielding H. Garrison, entitled "An epitome of the history of Spanish medicine," *Bulletin of the New York Academy of Medicine* (1931), 7:589–634.

2. For an overview of political, religious, and economic events, consult J.H. Elliott, *Imperial Spain 1469–1716* (New York: Mentor Bks., 1966); and Stanley G. Payne, *A History of Spain and Portugal*, 2 vols. (Madison: Univ. of Wisconsin Press, 1973), I, chs. 9–14.

3. Brief discussions of Renaissance epidemiology in Spain can be found in Luis S. Granjel, *Historia de la Medicina Española* (Barcelona: Sayma, 1962), 41; and L.S. Granjel and J. Riera Palmero, "Medicina y sociedad en la España renacentista," in *Historia Universal de la Medicina*, ed. Pedro Laín Entralgo (Barcelona: Salvat, 1973), IV:183–84.

4. For details, see B. Vincent, "La peste atlantica de 1596–1602," *Asclepio* (1976), 28:5–25. A general commentary concerning the plague epidemics is A. Carreras Panchón, "Las epidemias de peste en la España del Renacimiento," *Asclepio* (1977), 29:5–15. His article is followed by a number of other papers presented at the Fifth National Spanish Congress of Medical History, all papers dealing with the impact of epidemic disease in Spain from the sixteenth to nineteenth centuries.

5. For a good recent summary of this disease, see C. Shear Wood, "Syphilis in anthropological perspective," *Social Science and Medicine* (1978), *12*:47–55. See also F. Guerra, "The dispute over syphilis: Europe versus America," *Clio Medica* (1978), *13*:39–61.

6. See L.S. Granjel, "El ejercicio de la medicina en la sociedad española renacentista," *Cuadernos de Historia de la Medicina Española* (1971), *10*:13–53. More details can be obtained from the following monograph: Rafael Muñoz Garrido, *Ejercicio Legal de la Medicina en España - Siglos XV al XVIII* (Salamanca: Universidad de Salamanca, 1967).

7. L. García Ballester, "The minority of morisco physicians in Spain of the 16th century and their conflicts in a dominant Christian society," *Sudhoffs Archiv* (1976), *60*:211.

8. Documentation concerning several prominent empirics who offered their services to the Royal Court during the sixteenth and seventeenth centuries is contained in R. Munoz Garrido, "Empíricos sanitarios españos de los siglos XVI y XVII," *Cuad. Hist. Med. Esp.* (1967), *6*:101–33. The activities of the midwife are briefly summarized in C. Fernández Ruiz, "La comadrona en la historia de la obstetricia," *Gaceta Médica Española* (1955), *29*:462–65. For a description of the urban witch and her functions, consult L.S. Granjel, "Medicina y brujeria," *Cuad. Hist. Med. Esp.* (1972), *11*:407–20. See also M. Herrero, "Tipologia social del siglo XVII - ensalmadores y saludadores," *Hispania* (1955–56), *15*:173–90; and I. Yañez Polo and J.R. Zaragoza Rubira, "Spanish folk medicine of the XVIIth century," in *Acta Congressus Internationalis XXIV· Historiae Artis Medicinae* (Budapest: Semmelweis Museum, 1976), II:1287–93.

9. See Luis García Ballester, *Historia Social de la Medicina en la España de los Siglos XIII al XVI* (Madrid: Akal, 1976). There are very few secondary sources dealing with Jewish medicine in Spain, and those that do, concentrate on the accomplishments and writings of Moses ben Maimon (1135–1204) A chapter entitled "Jewish physicians in Spain and Portugal" appears in Aaron Friedenwald, *Jewish Physicians and the Contributions of the Jews to the Science of Medicine* (Philadelphia: Graetz College, 1897).

10. For more details, see Luis García Ballester, *Medicina, Ciencia y Minorias Marginadas: Los Moriscos* (Granada: Universidad de Granada, 1977).

11. For more details, see M. Parrilla Hermida, "Apuntes historicos sobre el protomedicato," *Anales de la Real Academia Nacional de Medicina—Madrid* (1977), *94*:475–515. For the background in Aragón, see also R. Jordi González and J.L. Gómez Camaño, "Mujeres y varones médicos por decision real en el reinado de Juan I de Aragón," *Boletín de la Sociedad Española de Historia de la Farmacia* (1968), *19*:145–52.

12. R. Roldán y Guerrero, "Los orígenes del tribunal del Real Proto-medicato de Castilla," *Archivo Iberoamericano de Historia de la Medicina* (1960), 12:249–54.

13. D. Vicente de la Fuente, *Historia de las Universidades, Colegios y demás Establecimientos de Enseñanza* (Madrid: Fuentenebro, 1885), esp. vol. 2, ch. 82, "Estado de los estudios de medicina en las principales universidades durante el siglo XVI," 472–81.

14. Luis Alonso Muñoyerro, *La Facultad de Medicina en la Universidad de Alcalá de Henares* (Madrid: Inst. Jerónimo Zurita, 1945), 27–29. For Granada, see J. Gutierrez Galdo, "Los planes de estudio de la facultad de medicina de Granada en los siglos XVI, XVII and XVIII," *Actualidad Medica* (1965), 41:643–55.

15. For a general panorama of Spanish medical education, see F. Guerra, "Medical education in Iberoamerica," in *The History of Medical Education*, ed. C.D. O'Malley (Berkeley: Univ. of California Press, 1970), 419–31.

16. Muñoyerro, 142.

17. Ibid., 91–94.

18. Ibid., 148–49.

19. Ibid., 150–52.

20. Ibid., 152–59.

21. Ibid., 160–75.

22. Ibid., 259–74, 291–92.

23. Ibid., 107–20.

24. For general background, see G. Rosen, "The hospital: historical sociology of a community institution," in *From Medical Police to Social Medicine: Essays on the History of Health Care* (New York: Science History Publications, 1974), 274–84.

25. T.S. Miller, "The Knights of Saint John and the hospitals of the Latin West," *Speculum* (1978), 53:709–33; and C. Probst, "Das Hospitalwesen in hohen und späten Mittelalter und die geistige und gesellschaftliche Stellung des Kranken," *Sudhoffs Archiv* (1966), 50:246–58.

26. M. Zuñiga Cisneros, "España, la medicina religiosa y los hospitales," *Archivo Iberoamer. Hist. Med.* (1956), 8:377–86. For a complete and detailed architectural analysis, see Dieter Jetter, *Geschichte des Hospitals: Spanien von den Anfängen bis um 1500* (Wiesbaden, Franz Steiner Verlag, 1980).

27. S. Hamarneh, "Development of hospitals in Islam," *Journal of the History of Medicine* (1962), 17:366–84, esp. 376–77.

28. G. Goldin, "Juan de Dios and the hospital of Christian charity," *J. Hist. Med.* (1978), 33:6–34. The quotation is from Juan Santos' history of St. John of God, *Chronología Hospitalaria y Resumen Historial de la Sagrada Religión del Glorioso Patriarca San Juan de Dios*, 2 vols. (Madrid, 1715), I:6.

29. See also the section on "Antecedentes historicos en la metropoli" in J. Guijarro Oliveras, "Historia de los hospitales coloniales españoles en America durante los siglos XVI, XVII y XVIII," *Archivo Iberoamer. Hist. Med.* (1950), 2:529–33. Some of these aims can also be detected in the pioneering Spanish treatment of the insane; see J.B. Ullersperger, *La Historia de la Psicología y de la Psiquiatría en España* (Madrid: Ed. Alhambra, 1954), and R.D. Clements, "The role of J.L. Vives in the development of modern medical science," unpubl. Ph.D. diss., Univ. of Chicago, 1964.

30. A brief summary of Spanish medical theory and practice in the Renaissance can be found in Granjel, *Historia de la Medicina Española*, 39–69; and J.M. López Piñero and F. Bujosa Homar, "Tradición y renovación de los saberes medicos en la España del siglo XVI," *Medicina Española* (1978), 77:355–66. For Valencia, see J.M. López Piñero, "Valencia y la medicina del Renacimiento y del Barroco," in *La Medicina, la Ciencia y la Técnica en la Historia Valenciana* (Madrid: Sociedad Española de Historia de la Medicina, 1971), 95–108.

31. For a more extensive list of the Hippocratic works published in this period, see Teresa Santander Rodriguez, *Hipócrates en España (Siglo XVI)* (Madrid: Dirección General de Archivos y Bibliotecas, 1971).

32. A useful and recent critical synthesis for this period is José M. López Piñero, *Ciencia y Técnica en la Sociedad Española de los Siglos XVI y XVII* (Barcelona: Editorial Labor, 1979), esp. the chapter "Los saberes medicos del galenismo arabizado al paracelsismo," 339–70.

33. J.M. López Piñero, "The Vesalian movement in sixteenth-century Spain," *Journal of the History of Biology* (1979), 12:45–81.

34. J.M. López Piñero and M.L. Terrada Ferrandiz, "La obra de Juan Tomas Porcell (1566) y los origenes de la anatomía patólogica moderna," *Med. Esp.* (1965), 53:237–50. A brief introduction to Porcell's work in English and excerpts from his influential work are contained in José M. López Piñero, Francesc Bujosa, and Maria Luz Terrada, *Clásicos Españoles de la Anatomía Patológica Anteriores a Cajal* (Valencia: Catedra e Instituto de Historia de la Medicina, 1979), 11–15, 60–67.

35. See also Luis S. Granjel, *Cirugía Española del Renacimiento* (Salamanca: Universidad de Salamanca, 1968).

36. G. Folch Jou, "Los médicos, la botánica y la materia médica farmacéutica en España durante la decimosexta centuria," *Asclepio* (1967), 19:141–55.

37. F.J. Pérez Fuenzalida, "Nicolás Monardes y Andrés Laguna: actitudes tradicionales y renovadoras en la medicina del Renacimiento," *Actas, IV Congreso Español de Historia de la Medicina* (Granada, 1973), I:73–79. For a more detailed study of Monardes, see E. Herrero Marcos,

"Vida y obra de Nicolás Monardes," *Cuad. Hist. Med. Esp.* (1962), 1:61–84.

38. R.S. Munger, "Guaiacum, the holy wood from the New World," *J. Hist. Med.* (1949), 4:196–229. For an overview of the drug traffic, see F. Guerra, "Drugs from the Indies and the political economy of the sixteenth century," *Analecta Medico Historica* (1966), 1:29–54.

39. J.M. López Piñero, "Paracelsus and his work in 16th and 17th century Spain," *Clio Medica* (1973), 8:113–14.

40. See George C. Vaillant, *Aztecs of Mexico: Origin, Rise, and Fall of the Aztec Nation,* 2nd ed. (New York: Penguin Books, 1965); and Jacques Soustelle, *Daily Life of the Aztecs on the Eve of the Spanish Conquest,* trans. P. O'Brian (Stanford, Calif.: Stanford Univ. Press, 1961).

41. The "Berkeley School" represented by Sherburne F. Cook and Woodrow Borah has provided the highest population estimates—25 million people—for central Mexico; "Conquest and population: a demographic approach to Mexican history," *Proceedings of the American Philosophical Society* (1969), 113:177–83. These figures have been drastically reduced by other authors; see, for example, W.T. Sanders, "The population of the Central Mexican symbiotic region, the basin of Mexico and the Teotihuacan Valley in the sixteenth century," in *The Native Population of the Americas in 1492,* ed. William M. Denevan (Madison: Univ. of Wisconsin Press, 1976), 85–150. Sanders allows for a total population of about 2.5 to 4.5 million people.

42. These figures come from Sanders, "The population of the Central Mexican symbiotic region," 148–49. For a recent estimate of the population, see R.A. Zambardino, "Mexico's population in the sixteenth century: demographic anomaly or mathematical illusion," *Journal of Interdisciplinary History* (1980), 11:1–27. The author estimated the 1518 population to be between 5 and 10 million people.

43. M.D. Coe, "The chinampas of Mexico," *Scientific American* (July 1964), 211:90–98. The use of a protein-rich alga, spirulina geitleri, as a staple of Aztec diets has also been recently discovered; see P.T. Furst, "Spirulina," *Human Nature* (March 1978), 1:60–65. For a summary of pre-Columbian foodstuffs, see E. Beltrán, "Plantas usadas en la alimentación por los antiguos Mexicanos," *America Indígena* (July 1949), 9:195–204; and E. Dávalos Hurtado, "La alimentación entre los Mexicas," *Revista Mexicana de Estudios Antropológicos* (1956), 14:103–18.

44. S.F. Cook, "The incidence and significance of disease among the Aztecs and related tribes," *Hispanic American Historical Review* (1946), 26:331–34. The idea of precarious food supplies in central Mexico has generated the assumption that Aztec cannibalism became a necessary custom to insure adequate protein supplies to the theocratic elite. See M.J. Harner, "The ecological basis for Aztec sacrifice," *American Ethnologist*

(1977), 4:117–35; and B.J. Price, "Demystification, enriddlement, and Aztec cannibalism: a materialist rejoinder to Harner," *American Ethnologist,* (1978), 5:98–115. This hypothesis has been categorically rejected by B.R. Ortiz de Montellano, "Aztec cannibalism: an ecological necessity?" *Science* (1978), 200:611–16, but a lively debate on this topic continues among anthropologists.

45. See P.M. Ashburn, *The Ranks of Death: A Medical History of the Conquest of America* (New York: Coward-McCann, 1947); Alfred W. Crosby, Jr., *The Columbian Exchange: Biological and Cultural Consequences of 1492* (Westport, Conn.: Greenwood, 1972).

46. T.D. Stewart, "A physical anthropologist's view of the peopling of the New World," *Southwest Journal of Anthropology* (1960), 16:259–73. For a discussion of this argument, see also M.T. Newman, "Aboriginal New World epidemiology and medical care, and the impact of Old World disease imports," *American Journal of Physical Anthropology* (1976), 45:667–72.

47. For an extensive discussion of this problem and its impact on historical events, see William H. McNeill, *Plagues and Peoples* (Garden City, N.Y.: Doubleday, 1976), esp. ch. V: "Transoceanic exchanges 1500–1700," 199–234.

48. See P.M. Newberne and G. Williams, "Nutritional influences on the course of infections," in *Resistance to Infectious Diseases,* ed. R.H. Dunlop and H.W. Moon (Saskatoon: Saskatoon Modern Press, 1970), 93–111.

49. For a list of the principal epidemics in New Spain between 1520 and 1800, see Charles Gibson, *The Aztecs under Spanish Rule* (Stanford, Calif.: Stanford Univ. Press, 1964), app. IV, 448–51.

50. F.L. Dunn, "On the antiquity of malaria in the Western hemisphere," *Human Biology* (1965), 37:383–93; and J. Friedlander, "Malaria and demography in the lowland of Mexico: an ethno-historical approach," *Proceedings of the American Ethnological Society* (Seattle: Univ. of Washington Press, 1969), 217–33.

51. This disease prompted a Spanish physician, Francisco Hernández, to write a small unpublished monograph about its clinical symptoms, supplemented by autopsy findings; see G. Somolinos D'Ardois, "Hallazgo del manuscripto sobre el cocoliztli original del Dr. Francisco Hernández," *La Prensa Médica Mexicana* (Sept.–Dec. 1956), 21:115–22. The nature of the disease remains shrouded in mystery and periodically tempts physicians to diagnose it retroactively on the basis of modern medical knowledge.

52. An excellent case study about conditions in Cholula and the synchronism of malnutrition and infection is E. Malvido, "Efectos de las epidemias y hambrunas en la población colonial de Mexico," *Salud Pública de México,* Epoca V (Nov.-Dec. 1975), 17:793–802.

53. See C.W. Goff, "New evidence of pre-Columbian bone syphilis in Guatemala," in *The Rivers of Zacculeu, Guatemala,* ed. R.B. Woodbury (Richmond, Va.: Byrd Press, 1953), 312–19; and N.G. Gejvall and F. Henschen, "Anatomical evidence of pre-Columbian syphilis in the West Indian Islands," *Beiträge der Pathologie* (1971), *144:*138–57.

54. L. Marquez de González, "Disease and society in colonial Mexico: the skeletons from the National Cathedral," *Paleopathology Newsletter* (Dec. 1980), *32:*608.

55. Cortés commented about the abundance of healing herbs. See J. Bayard Morris, trans., *Hernando Cortés — Five Letters, 1519–1526* (New York: Norton, n.d.), 51. See also T. Motolinia, *History of the Indians of New Spain,* trans. and ed. E.A. Foster (Berkeley, Calif.: Cortes Society, 1950), 211.

56. For details, see Francisco Fernández del Castillo and Alicia Hernandez Torres, *El Tribunal del Protomedicato en la Nueva España, según el Archivo Histórico de la Facultad de Medicina* (Mexico: U.N.A.M., 1965). John Tate Lanning's important history of *The Royal Protomedicato: The Regulation of the Medical Professions in the Spanish Empire,* ed. John J. TePaske (Durham, N.C.: Duke Univ. Press, 1985) unfortunately appeared too late to be used in this study. A brief survey in English is R.M. Price, "The protomedicato in New Spain," *International Symposium on Society, Medicine and Law,* ed H. Karplus (Amsterdam: Elsevier Scientific Publications, 1973), 77–89. Price has recently written a more extensive paper, "The protomedicatos of the Spanish empire," for the International symposium at the University of Valencia, Spain, 15–17 Dec. 1980, entitled "Factors in the Diffusion of Science Across Cultural Frontiers."

57. J.T. Lanning, "Legitimacy and *Limpieza de Sangre* in the practice of medicine in the Spanish empire," *Jahrbuch fuer Geschichte von Staat, Wirtschaft, und Gesellschaft Lateinamerikas* (1967), *4:*37–60.

58. J.T. Lanning, "The illicit practice of medicine in the Spanish empire in America," in *Homenaje a Don José María de la Peña y Cámara,* ed. Ernest J. Burros (Madrid: Ed. J. Porrua Turanzas, 1969), 150.

59. Castillo and Torres, *Tribunal del Protomedicato,* 14–15.

60. See Manuel Soriano, "Algunos apuntes sobre el protomedicato," *Gaceta médica Mexicana* (1899), *36:*563–89; and John T. Lanning, *The Eighteenth Century Enlightenment in the University of San Carlos de Guatemala* (Ithaca, N.Y.: Cornell Univ. Press, 1956), esp. 222–63.

61. For an overview of Hernández' life and activities, see Germán Somolinos D'Ardois, *El Doctor Francisco Hernández y la Primera Expedición Científica en América* (Mexico: Secretaria de Educacion Publica, 1971). For more detail, see the same author's *Vida y Obra de Francisco Hernández* (Mexico: Universidad Nacional de Mexico, 1960), 160–93.

62. The story has been masterfully reconstructed by John T. Lanning in his book *Pedro de la Torre: Doctor to Conquerors* (Baton Rouge: Louisiana State Univ. Press, 1974).

63. Ibid., 6–22.

64. J.M. Reyes, "Estudios históricos sobre el ejercicio de la medicina 1646–1800," *Anales de la Escuela de Medicina* (Mexico, 1912), 1:511–73.

65. This subject has received a great deal of attention. The best book, Gonzalo Aguirre Beltrán, *Medicina y Magia* (Mexico: Instituto Nacional Indigenista, 1963), combines historical and anthropological perspectives.

66. *Recopilación de Leyes de los Reynos de las Indias*, 4 vols. (Madrid, 1681). A recent reprint of this collection of documents has been used (Madrid: Ed. Cultura Hispánica, 1973), II: 159.

67. For more details, see Alberto Maria Carreño, *La Real y Pontificia Universidad de Mexico 1536–1835* (Mexico: Universidad Nacional Autónoma de Mexico, 1961).

68. The most complete description of medical education in colonial Mexico is contained in a series of articles written by Nicolás León entitled: "Apuntes para la historia de la enseñanza y ejercicio de la medicina en Mexico desde la conquista hispana hasta el año de 1833." The early period, 1521–82, appeared in *Gac. méd. Mex.*, 3a serie (1915), 10:466–89. The others appeared in 1918, 11:210–86, and 1921, 55:3–48.

69. Ibid., 470–74. The original document was reprinted in Francisco Fernández del Castillo, *La Facultad de Medicina según el Archivo de la Real y Pontificia Universidad de Mexico* (Mexico: Consejo de Humanidades, 1953), 83–85.

70. See Guerra, "Medical education in Iberoamerica," 432–34. Greater detail is available in A.M. Rodríguez Cruz, *Historia de las Universidades Hispanoamericanas: Periodo Hispanico*, 2 vols. (Bogota: Inst. Caro y Cuervo, 1973).

71. The data, seemingly based on original documents, were obtained from the yearly list of graduates in León, "Apuntes para la historia de la enseñanza." For the period 1582–1600, consult *Gac. méd. Mex.*, 3a série (1918), 11:212–15.

72. See Julio Jiménez Rueda, *Historia de la Cultura en Mexico: El Virreinato* (Mexico: Ed. Cultura, 1950), 271–77; and Tomas Zepeda Rincón, *La Instrucción Pública en la Nueva España en el Siglo XVI* (Mexico: Univ. Nac. Mex., 1933), 99–116. See also Guillermo S. Fernández de Recas, *Medicina: Nómina de bachilleres, licenciados y doctores 1607–1780 y guia de méritos y servicios 1763–1828* (*Real y Pontificia Universidad de Mexico*) (Mexico: U.N.A.M., 1960).

73. Fernández del Castillo, *La Facultad de Medicina*, 15–19, 110–13.

74. Ibid., 114–42.

75. J. Guijarro Oliveras, "Política sanataria en las Leyes de Indias," *Archivo Iberoamer. Hist. Med.* (1957), 9:255–62.

76. Both education and hospitals were largely under the control of the Church as divisions of the Real Patronato de Indias. See John L. Mecham, "Church and state during the Spanish regime in America," in *Church and State in Latin America*, rev. ed. (Chapel Hill: Univ. of North Carolina Press, 1966), 3–37.

77. *Cartas de Indias*, No. 8 (Madrid, 1877), p. 52, as quoted in Robert Ricard, *The Spiritual Conquest of Mexico*, trans. L. Byrd Simpson (Berkeley: Univ. of California Press, 1966), 350.

78. Ibid., pp. 155–61. For a summary of the influence exerted by the Church, see F. Guerra, "The role of religion in Spanish American medicine," in *Medicine and Culture*, ed. F.N.L. Poynter (London: Wellcome Institute, 1969), 179–88. For an overview of institutional development in New Spain, see Colin M. MacLachlan and Jaime E. Rodríguez O., "The institutional process," in *The Forging of the Cosmic Race* (Berkeley: Univ. of California Press, 1980), ch. 5, pp. 95–143.

79. W. Borah, "Social welfare and social obligation in New Spain: a tentative assessment," *Proceedings, International Congress of Americanists* (1966), no. 4, 36:45–57. See also J. Guijarro Oliveras, "Caracteres comunes de las instituciones nosocomiales coloniales españolas en América," *Archivo Iberoamer. Hist. Med.* (1950), 2:594–99.

80. For the original documents, see Diego de Encinas, *Cedulario Indiano*, 4 vols. (1596; rpt. Madrid: Ed. Cultura Hispánica, 1945), vol. I, folio 219. According to Mecham, *Church and State in Latin America*, Encinas' collection of documents is more extensive than the often-quoted *Recopilación de Leyes de los Reynos de las Indias* of 1681.

81. Josefina Muriel, "Hospital de la Concepción de Nuestra Señora," in *Hospitales de la Nueva España;* 2 vols. (Mexico: Ed. Jus, 1956–60), I:36–48.

82. See Robert Richard, *Etudes et documents pour l'histoire missionnaire de l'Espagne et du Portugal* (Louvain, A.U.C.A.M.–E. Desbarax, 1931), 85.

83. See also Muriel, *Hospitales de la Nueva España;* J. Guijarro Oliveras, "Historia de los hospitales coloniales españoles en América durante los siglos XVI, XVII y XVIII," *Archivo Iberoamer. Hist. Med.* (1950), 2:529–93. An overview of hospitals for the mentally ill is provided by C. Viqueira, "Los hospitales para locos e inocentes en Hispanoamerica y sus antecedentes españoles," *Revista Española de Antropología Americana* (1970), 5:341–84. More detail is available in Juan Delgado Roig, *Fundaciones Psiquiátricas en Sevilla y Nuevo Mundo* (Madrid: Ed. Paz Montalvo, 1948).

84. For a brief summary, see C. Venegas Ramírez, "La asistencia hospitalaria para Indios en la Nueva España," *Anales Instituto de Antropologia e Historia* (1966), 19:227–40. See also David A. Howard, *The Royal Indian Hospital of Mexico City* (Tempe: Center for Latin American Studies, Arizona State Univ., 1980), 1–10, which deals with the history of the hospital during the eighteenth and early nineteenth centuries.

85. See also Carmen Venegas Ramírez, *Régimen Hospitalario para Indios en la Nueva España* (Mexico: Inst. Nac. Antrop. Hist., 1973).

86. J. Somolinos, "De los hospitals de la Nueva España, un legado que se pierde," *Gac. méd. Mex.* (1976), 112:449–58.

87. Somolinos D'Ardois, *Vida y Obra Hernández*, 202–204.

88. M.M. Lucas, "A social welfare organizer in New Spain: Don Vasco de Quiroga, first bishop of Michoacán," *The Americas* (1957), 14.57–86.

89. J. Muriel, *Hospitales,* I: 55–64.

90. See also Fintan B. Warren, *Vasco de Quiroga and his Pueblo-Hospitals of Santa Fe* (Washington, D.C.: Acad. Amer. Franciscan Hist., 1963).

91. Mariano Cuevas, *Documentos Inéditos del Siglo XVI para la Historia de Mexico* (Mexico, 1914), 328, as quoted in Ricard, *The Spiritual Conquest of Mexico,* 156.

92. For a detailed analysis of the *cofradías,* their organization, and function, see Adolfo Lamas, *Seguridad Social en la Nueva España* (Mexico: U.N.A.M., 1964), ch. III, 126–58.

93. See *Recopilación de Leyes de los Reynos de las Indias,* II, folio 159.

94. C.H. Talbot, "America and the European drug trade," in *First Images of America,* ed. Fredi Chiappelli, 2 vols. (Berkeley: Univ. of California Press, 1976), II:833–44.

95. For an interesting analysis of the empirical effectiveness of Aztec drugs, see B. Ortiz de Montellano, "Empirical Aztec medicine," *Science* (18 April 1975), 188:215–20. Most Spanish chroniclers reported on native health conditions and healing practices, see J.L. Gómez Ratón, "Capítulos médicos en la obra de los historiadores de Indias" *Cuad. Hist. Med. Esp.* (1963), 2:43–80.

96. Emily Walcott Emmart, *The Badianus Manuscript* (Baltimore: John Hopkins Press, 1940). See also Emmart, "An Aztec medical treatise, the Badianus manuscript," *Bulletin of the Institute of the History of Medicine* (1935), 3:483–506. More recent scholarship can be found in E.C. del Pozo, "Symposium sobre el códice de medicina Azteca de Martín de la Cruz y Juan Badiano," *Gac. méd. Mex.* (1964), 94:115–120.

97. Somolinos D'Ardois, *Vida y Obra de Hernández,* 194–224.

98. Ibid., 174–78, 400–402. Hernández' work has been translated into Spanish by J. Garcia Pimentel, *Antiguedades de la Nueva España*

(Mexico: Ed. Pedro Robredo, 1945). For a translation of Hernández' treatise on the cocoliztli, see G. Somolinos D'Ardois, "Hallazgo del manuscripto sobre el cocoliztli, original del Dr. Francisco Hernandez," *La Prensa Médica Mexicana* (Sept.–Dec. 1956), 21:115–22.

99. For a summary of the Aztec herbs and their actions, see E.C. del Pozo, "Aztec pharmacology," *Annual Review of Pharmacology* (1966), 6:9–18. A more extensive treatment of the subject by the same author is "La botánica medicinal indígena de Mexico," *Estudios de Cultura Nahautl* (1965), 5:57–73.

100. A good summary of early Mexican medical authors and their works is G. Somolinos D'Ardois, "Médicos y libros en el primer siglo de la colonia," *Boletín de la Biblioteca Nacional* (Mexico, 1967), 18:99–137. Information on Francisco Bravo is contained in Francisco Guerra's introduction to Bravo's *The Opera Medicinalia* (London: Dawsons, 1970). See also the extensive and informative review of this reprint by S. Jarcho, *Bulletin of the History of Medicine* (1972), 46:195–98.

101. G. Somolinos D'Ardois, "Francisco Bravo y su 'Opera Medicinalia'" *Anales de la Sociedad Médica de Historia de la Ciencia y Tecnología* (1970), 2:117–45.

102. S. Jarcho, "Medicine in sixteenth-century New Spain as illustrated by the writings of Bravo, Farfán, and Vargas Machuca," *Bull. Hist. Med.* (1957), 31:427–31.

103. G. Somolinos D'Ardois, "El cirujano López de Hinojosos, su obra quirurgica, y la companía de Jesús," in *La Companía de Jesús en México: Cuatro Siglos de Labor Cultural* (Mexico, 1972), 525–76.

104. Alonso López de Hinojosos, *Suma y Recopilación de Cirugia* (1578; rpt. Mexico: Academia Nacional de Medicina, 1977), 77. The work contains a brief introduction written by G. Somolinos D'Ardois.

105. Ibid., 207–13.

106. See N. Quezada, "La herbolaria en el Mexico colonial," in *Estado Actual del Conocimiento en Plantas Medicinales Mexicanas,* ed X. Lozoya (Mexico: Instituto Mexicano para el Estudio de las Plantas Medicinales, 1978), 51–68. See also C. Viesca Treviño, "Alonso López y su Suma y Recopilación de Cirugia, 1535–1597," in *Estudios sobre Ethnobotánica y Antropología Médica,* ed. C. Viesca Treviño (Mexico: Instituto Mexicano para el Estudio de las Plantas Medicinales, 1976), 29–58.

107. See Jarcho, "Medicine in sixteenth century New Spain," 431–39; and J. Comas, "Influencia indígena en la medicina hipocrática en la Nueva España del Siglo XVI," *America Indígena* (1954), 14:327–61.

108. Agustín Farfán, *Tractado Breve de Medicina* (1592; rpt. Madrid: Ed. Cultura Hispánica, 1944), folio 1.

109. Ibid., folio 41.

110. J. Comas, "Influencia de la medicina Azteca en la obra de Fr.

Agustín Farfán," *Proceedings, International Congress of Americanists* (1955), 31:27–30; and G. Folch Jou, "Las drogas en la obra de Fray Agustín Farfán," *Actas, Internacional Congreso de Historia de la Medicina* (Madrid, 1956), II: 165–81.

111. See Germán Somolinos D'Ardois, *El Fenómeno de Fusión Cultural y su Trascendencia Médica: Capítulos de Historia Médica Mexicana II* (Mexico, 1979).

2

Medicine in New France

Toby Gelfand

> . . . in the various nations, medical theory is enclosed
> within the confines of familiar practices, supported by
> popular prejudices and sustained and perpetuated by
> the example and authority of the most sought-after
> practitioners.
> —François Quesnay, *Essai physique sur l'économie animale* (Paris, 1747), vol. 1, p. lxvii

Medicine in the New World presents the historian with a "natural experiment" for testing the effect of a new environment on the transmission of European beliefs and practices. In the case of New France, a colony that began with the explorations of Jacques Cartier in the 1530s and came to an abrupt termination with the British conquest two and one-third centuries later, medical structures were clearly derived from the mother country. At the same time, they bore the imprint of the colony's radically different natural and economic conditions. In what follows, I shall first sketch the disease situation and the organization of medicine in seventeenth- and eighteenth-century France under the Old Regime in order to provide background for a more extended comparison with medicine in the New France colony.

MEDICINE IN FRANCE

At the outset of the eighteenth century, France was easily the most populous country in Western Europe. With about twenty million inhabitants, a total that had remained fairly constant for several centuries, the France of Louis XIV appeared as the preeminent agricultural, commercial, and military power of the period. Great Britain, France's major rival in building and contesting a colonial empire, drew on a population of only nine million.[1]

From about 1740, the French population began to increase, attaining about twenty-five million by the end of the century. The causes of this demographic expansion remain obscure. Better nutrition, living conditions, transportation, and possibly even general medical attention, if not specific treatments for disease, contributed, but there were other factors. For example, the proliferation of foundling hospitals for abandoned infants during this period (despite their appalling rates of mortality) witnessed a basic shift in collective attitudes toward those who might earlier have been victims of infanticide. For whatever reasons, the period after about midcentury in France saw a transformation of the age-old pattern of periodic massive famines leaving economic crises and epidemics in their wakes. These kinds of demographic catastrophes gave way to an irregular pattern of isolated epidemics, which usually did not produce the levels of mortality common in earlier centuries.

France had an overwhelmingly rural population. About 85 percent of the inhabitants, almost all of whom were peasants, lived in villages and countryside. Yet, there were important cities, the great capital Paris, of course, with about a half-million inhabitants constituted (with its appendage, Versailles) the political, commercial, and cultural hub of an increasingly centralized state. Seven other cities counted populations between 50,000 and 100,000, including the commercial center, Lyons, and the port cities of Marseilles and Bordeaux. Some sixty other towns had more than 10,000 inhabitants. Thus France's population had a significant and, during the eighteenth century, a growing urban component.

Pattern of Diseases

Any attempt to determine the identity and frequency of diseases during the early modern period inevitably founders on several methodological problems. Sources are sparse and scattered. Medical observers seldom had the resources or disposition to report diseases in quantitative terms prior to the nineteenth century. Finally, and perhaps most perplexing, it is often difficult to state precisely or with confidence the modern disease entities to which the old medical descriptions might correspond. How can one translate 128 different kinds of fevers mentioned in eighteenth-century texts into modern equivalents?[2] Obviously the historian is thwarted by the fact that older medical classifications, lacking anatomical and causal systems for defining diseases, differed fundamentally from those accepted today. Furthermore, sick people in early modern times commonly suffered from malnutrition and various mixtures of chronic deficiencies and secondary infections that make their ailments difficult to diagnose in modern times.

Nevertheless, it seems safe to say (and the sources suggest) that inhabitants of Old Regime France suffered from the following maladies nearly every year in varying degrees of severity and occasionally at epidemic levels: serious lung diseases, especially pneumonia; gastrointestinal disorders, especially dysentery; typhoid and typhus, malaria, and smallpox. Also present in endemic and, occasionally, epidemic form were scurvy and diseases resulting from surgical or obstetrical infections such as "hospital gangrene" and puerperal fever respectively. Finally, there was a host of non-epidemic yet widespread ailments, including congenital malformations, rickets, gout, stone of the bladder, and many others.[3]

It remains a moot question whether conditions of health were worse in city or countryside, though the traditional viewpoint that cities were more dangerous seems to stand. Certainly, the cities had more extensive medical services, personnel, and institutions and therefore did a better job of documenting their diseases. Cases of tuberculosis, for example, were seldom identified in the countryside, though they probably were not uncommon.[4] Epidemics of pneumonia might well wreak greater havoc upon an isolated village lacking food and other supplies than upon a city possessing such amenities. In either case, wretched local living conditions (food, clothing, shelter, sanitation) largely determined the extent of mortality in any given epidemic. In addition to such material stresses, it has been suggested that a precarious collective psychology among rural masses accounts for a widespread occurrence of convulsions and other mental symptoms as complications of somatic illness or as independent phenomena.[5]

A study of the reigning pathological conditions in Lyons during the seventeenth and eighteenth centuries provides a representative sample of diseases in the urban setting.[6] Certain epidemics of the medieval and Renaissance periods, like leprosy and ergotism, disappeared entirely. Bubonic plague, a recurrent terror through the early seventeenth century, also ceased to strike Lyons; the last major outbreak in France, the plague of Marseilles (1720) remained confined to the southern provinces. Although Lyons suffered from all the infectious diseases enumerated above—typhoid was common in the autumn season when rivers overflowed into wells or, alternatively, in the summer when riverbeds dried up—the eighteenth century situation has been characterized by one historian as an "improvement" when compared with the "tragic" seventeenth century.[7] Smallpox, for example, previously a dangerous epidemic striking the entire population, settled down into an endemic pattern largely confined to children

Organization of Medical Practice

The organization of medical practice in Old Regime France consisted of a complicated patchwork of conflicting corporate bodies, private initiatives, local municipal arrangements, and government regulations. In principle, the three organized groups concerned with medicine—physicians, surgeons, and apothecaries—were unified insofar as physicians alone had the legal right to practice the healing art. Surgeons and apothecaries were simply to follow the physicians' commands in their appropriate subordinate tasks, the treatment of "external" or surgical ailments and the preparation of drugs respectively.[8]

Physicians as a group formed corporative bodies or faculties of medicine that, along with theology and law, constituted the higher faculties of universities. In France there were some twenty-two medical faculties, of which Paris and Montpellier were the most important. Others, such as Rheims in Champagne or Pont-à-Mousson in Lorraine, were little more than "degree mills" or places where a medical degree might easily be acquired after a short residence, or even in absentia, provided the candidate could pay the necessary fees. In principle, medical education involved many years of study during which the prospective physician, already in possession of an arts degree from a university, attended medical courses, passed a series of oral and written examinations, and sustained various theses. All this work was conducted in the Latin language, and there was no provision for practical training until the medical student had passed the stages of bachelor and licentiate. At that point, after perhaps six years, a brief period with an older practitioner or some hospital experience would precede the conferring of the doctorate in a lavish ceremony to the considerable financial expense of the candidate.

Medical faculties thus controlled the teaching, examining, and licensing of physicians; they also served as professional guilds with a vested interest in protecting their members' monopoly over medical practice and their privileged status in society.

The jurisdiction of the medical faculties extended, in principle, to include authority over the guilds of apothecaries and barber-surgeons. Physicians, acting as representatives of the Paris faculty, offered special courses in French in pharmacy and surgical operations to apprentices and journeymen from the respective Paris guilds. Physicians also had the legal right to preside over the examinations of new masters to the guilds of surgeons and apothecaries, both of which rendered symbolic and financial homage to the medical faculty in annual ceremonies. In practice, the unity of the medical profession along hierarchical lines was seldom realized. Outside of the households of royalty and the great nobility, few patients could afford the luxury of simultaneously employing physicians, surgeons, and apothecaries. Most people in cities as well as rural areas were more likely to consult surgeons or apothecaries rather than physicians for their medical needs.

In effect, surgeons were the ordinary practitioners of medicine. This was primarily because common people, to the extent that they could or wished to pay for medical services, could only afford humble practitioners. Second, a sort of social congruence between practitioner and patient obtained for surgeons, most of whom had the status of artisans. Physicians, on the other hand, as liberal professionals, were socially removed from the majority of the patient population. To a lesser extent, this was also the case with apothecaries, who tended to be rather well-to-do merchants. Finally, surgeons predominated because the basic stock-in-trade of their practice was phlebotomy or blood letting by cutting open veins with a lancet. Phlebotomy, abetted by a few other fairly simple modes of treatment, such as purgation, found employment in nearly all diseases. Thus, from a technical standpoint, surgeons were perceived as usually necessary and often sufficient.

As a result of these factors, surgeons greatly outnumbered physicians (and apothecaries) in French towns. At Paris and Lyons, there were at least three times as many master surgeons as physicians, and an even greater proportion if one counts inferior grades of surgeons. A Lyons doctor complained that surgeons collectively received 90 percent of the revenues paid for the practice of internal medicine. Very few doctors of medicine lived in the countryside; in an area around Toulouse that included some 200 villages, there were only 8 physicians but 101 surgeons and 134 midwives. The diocese of Auch-en-Gascogne, whose almost entirely rural population of 60,000 roughly equalled that of New France, licensed more than 200 surgeons during the last twenty years of the Old Regime. The French countryside thus was not lacking in ordinary practitioners of medicine.[2]

Indeed the main reason for this profusion of country practitioners was their very mediocrity. Paris, of course, had several dozen highly skilled surgeons who did major operations, and there were smaller groups in the other cities who, during the eighteenth century, began to pursue liberal studies and achieve a status comparable with medical doctors. But this surgical elite made up a very small proportion of the legally recognized surgeons.

The typical village surgeon began to learn his craft during a two- or three-year apprenticeship, in many instances working under his own father. After apprenticeship, the surgical journeyman then entered a period of further practical training which might last many years and involve extensive travel throughout France or even Europe and the overseas colonies. Some entered military and naval service and gained experience in hospitals. During the eighteenth century, especially after 1750, surgical journeymen included courses of study at royal colleges of surgery at Paris (founded

1724) and at those newly established in provincial centers such as Rouen, Lyons, Montpellier, Bordeaux, and Toulouse.

The surgeon might eventually seek to qualify as a "master." If he had traveled during his years as a journeyman, he now typically returned to his home region and applied to the nearest town with a surgical community or guild. By this stage, he might well be in his thirties or even older. There were three levels of master surgeon; the lowest, and the one that the vast majority of aspirants sought, demanded a single three-hour examination on phlebotomy and the rudiments of surgery. If successful, the new master became legally entitled to perform a limited number of simple surgical procedures within the confines of a given village and its environs.

Many, if not most, surgical careers never advanced even to this lowest level of licensure by one of the hundreds of guilds scattered across France. These surgical guilds or "communities" were legally recognized professional companies that included all the master surgeons residing in a given town. Their statutes, granted by the royal government, gave them jurisdiction over examining, licensing, and regulating practitioners in the town and surrounding region. Those who did not qualify as masters might nonetheless practice by means of a variety of quasi-legal mechanisms provided by the guild, for example, as so-called "experts" licensed for a "specialty," like bone-setting, tooth-pulling, or applying trusses to hernias. The surgical guild also licensed midwives and thus claimed surveillance over large numbers of women who sometimes practiced medicine in addition to their formally defined role.[10]

Other healers practiced their art outside the guild structure, some by means of a "privilege" conferred by local officials, others as part of the duties traditionally assumed by parish priests and certain religious healing orders such as the Augustinian nursing sisters of the Hôtel-Dieu hospitals and the brothers of Saint-Jean-de-Dieu, who practiced medicine and surgery in several dozen Charité hospitals in France and the colonies. Still others—journeymen surgeons, local artisans, traveling drug vendors, shepherds, and blacksmiths—simply became self-styled healers. From the perspective of the surgical guilds, all of these unofficial healers came under the pejorative heading of "charlatans" or "empiricks."[11]

In terms of medical practice, no sharp barrier separated the world of official from unofficial medicine. The medical professions of Old Regime France appeared rather like a pyramid in structure, a pyramid that mirrored the enveloping society. At the top perched relatively few physicians and a surgical elite, who made considerable scientific and social progress during the eighteenth century. As one descended the pyramid, the number of practitioners expanded rapidly to accommodate widening geographical and social niches. Apothecaries and an elaborate hierarchy of surgeons gradually merged into midwives, quasi-legal, and illegal practitioners. Nevertheless, substantial numbers of sick poor were doubtless unable to afford access even to the lower reaches of this network of private practitioners. At the same time, the vast majority of practitioners must have had difficulties earning a living exclusively by treating the sick; hence combined occupations such as barber-surgeon, innkeeper-surgeon, and apothecary-spicer were the rule.

A variety of public or collective measures, some local and others central, addressed themselves to gaps in the system sketched above. An enormous network of nearly 2,000 charity hospitals ramified throughout eighteenth-century France.[12] Most had small capacities of ten or fewer beds and depended on the church for their meager support and staffing. Large general hospitals (Hôpitaux-Généraux) founded by the French Crown from the middle of the seventeenth century had more to do with the repression of poverty by means of incarceration than the treatment of the sick. The Hôtels-Dieu, which were intended for the treatment of the sick, often evoked fear and with good reason; the mortality of some, like the dreaded Hôtel-Dieu of Paris, tended to be very high. Yet they served as last resorts for the sick poor. And the larger hospitals, supported by the Crown and local governments and run by secular administrators, provided salaried posts for some physicians and many more surgeons.

In many instances, small towns contracted with physicians or surgeons to assure the presence of competent medical care. Public or municipal medical officers received stipends in return for treating the poor gratis, but medical men demanded fees from those who could afford to pay. Another type of contractual arrangement saw groups of families retain medical services

over a specified period by payment in advance.[13] In cities, medical officers held various salaried posts in public institutions—pris-
ons, courts, hospitals, monasteries, seminaries, etc.—and as
members of the entourage of public officials. The extended royal
household at Versailles employed several hundred salaried medical officers. The king's premier surgeon sold offices to provincial surgeons in towns throughout France. In exchange for local
responsibility for organizing surgeons, such posts conferred
financial and social advantages on the purchasers.[14]

Finally, as the eighteenth century progressed, the central government devoted increasing energy and funds to problems of
epidemic diseases among humans and animals. The founding
of a medical society in 1776, the Société Royale de Médecine,
marked the culmination of this campaign.[15] Many of the provincial correspondents of the Société had already served for years
as so-called royal "epidemic" physicians or surgeons, employed
by the government to organize a sanitary and medical response
to epidemics. The French government had acted in this manner
to mobilize medical personnel in Paris and the southern provinces at the time of the plague of 1720. From the early eighteenth
century, the office of controller general also funded the distribution of boxes of remedies to provincial centers, where they were
forwarded to local parish priests and others who treated the
poor.[16]

Medical Theory and Practice

The Paris medical faculty, as the official arbiter of proper
medical theory, adhered to a conservative tradition ultimately
derived from the authority of the ancient physician Galen. In
the name of Galenism, the faculty resisted for more than a half-
century the new physiology based upon William Harvey's discovery in the 1620s of the circulation of the blood. Notions of
pathology did not deviate substantially from the ancient concept of an equilibrium of the four humors. Hygiene remained
primarily a matter of the individual's responsibility to live tem-
perately and thereby maintain a balance of the so-called "non-
naturals" or environmental factors (for example, food, air, and
sleep) that influenced health.[17]

In keeping with ancient wisdom, therapy was directed at the whole person, who was viewed as an integrated dynamic system rather than as a collection of anatomically distinct organs. Thus phlebotomy and other evacuating remedies aimed to restore equilibrium by reducing an excess or simply by shifting body fluids away from the affected area. Blistering and various counter-irritants operated on the same principle. Herbal remedies were favored over inorganic substances as being more "natural"; hence the faculty bitterly opposed the introduction of the mineral antimony as a cathartic in the mid-seventeenth century.

The only effective challenge to the dogmatism of the Paris medical faculty came from the faculty at Montpellier in the south of France. Its own venerable tradition, its popularity as a school, and the success of its graduates in finding medical posts at the royal court gave Montpellier considerable prestige throughout Europe. Antimony, for example, successfully entered French medical practice via Montpellier and the royal connection. Whereas Paris medical thought in the early eighteenth century tended to be influenced by mechanistic notions, such as comparing the body to a hydraulic machine, Montpellier physicians championed a vitalistic interpretation, which stressed the unique properties of living matter.[18]

The Hippocratic revival that came to characterize French medical thought in general by the second half of the eighteenth century probably had its sources at Montpellier. Besides insisting that living or vital processes could not be reduced to physical or chemical activities, the Hippocratic approach encouraged clinical observation at the bedside. This fit in with renewed interest in hospital medicine and case histories. Following and greatly expanding the precedent of the seventeenth-century "English Hippocrates," Thomas Sydenham, progressive French physicians of the second half of the eighteenth century related diseases to weather patterns, soil, geological features, and demographic characteristics. The ultimate goal was a medical topography of the kingdom that would lead to an understanding of the "natural history" of diseases and eventually permit prediction and rational control of epidemics.[19]

While seldom in blatant contradiction with the theories sketched above, the practice of medicine, to the extent that it is known, seems to have been governed more by practical and empirical than theoretical concerns. Yet there were correlations between the two. French medical men apparently did tend to employ more aggressive bleeding and purging than their neighbors, and Jean Baptiste Molière's caricatures thus had some basis in reality.[20] Inoculation for the prevention of smallpox did not find acceptance in France until nearly a half-century later than England, in part because of the Paris faculty's objections.[21]

With the Hippocratic revival, enlightened French physicians began to adopt a more "expectant" or wait-and-see attitude toward therapy. The use of cinchona bark to treat fevers and mercurial compounds for venereal diseases formed part of standard medical practice throughout Europe. French surgical and obstetrical techniques made their practitioners undisputed leaders in these fields down through the first half of the eighteenth century.[22]

NEW FRANCE

After Jacques Cartier's initial voyages of exploration to the Saint Lawrence Valley in the 1530s, it took nearly a century for the French to establish a permanent colony in the New World. Samuel de Champlain founded Quebec in 1608, and Montreal was not settled until 1642. In the 1660s, New France counted only about 3,000 European inhabitants, of whom about two-thirds lived in the region around the town of Quebec. Approximately two-thirds of the population were rural-based, a proportion somewhat lower than in the mother country. But New France never supported any cities. Neither of the two main towns, Quebec and Montreal, acquired as many as 10,000 inhabitants during the French regime, and Trois-Rivières remained scarcely more than a large village. On the eve of the British conquest in 1760 perhaps one-fourth of the population lived in towns, of which Quebec, with just under 8,000 persons, was the largest.[23]

Thus the undeniable demographic reality of New France was a tiny population scattered over an immense territory extending from the Atlantic Coast to the Great Lakes and south along the Mississippi to the Gulf of Mexico. The vast majority of the settlers were concentrated in the Canadian colony in the Saint Law-

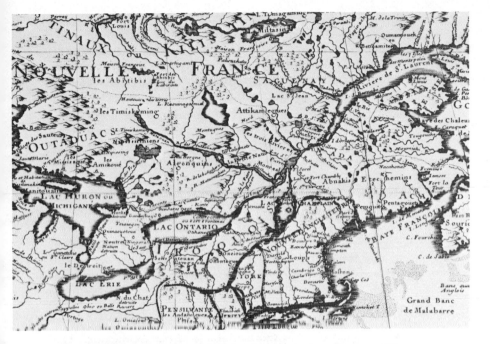

Detail from a map of New France showing the Saint Lawrence River
Valley and major settlements at Quebec City and Montreal. Carte
du Canada et de la Nouvelle France by Guillaume Delisle, Paris,
1703; from a facsimile produced by the Association of Canadian
Map Libraries, Queen's University, Kingston, Ontario.

rence River Valley. Although the population of this colony increased briskly during the eighteenth century, from about 15,000 to 76,000 at the time of the conquest, the increase was due largely to a remarkably high birth rate (nearly 60 per 1,000) rather than to immigration, which was modest. During the entire colonial period a total of only about 10,000 immigrants settled in New France; during the seventeenth century the average was only twenty per year. As a consequence, New France appeared miniscule compared with the British colonies, never exceeding more than about one-twentieth the combined population of its neighbors to the south.

Another condition limiting colonial development was the harsh northern climate. This made for a short growing season in a soil none too arable in the first place. Communication with the mother country halted during six months of the year, and given the transit time of two to three months, settlers could not expect more than one arrival from France each year. Lacking the means to supply themselves, the people of New France remained extraordinarily dependent on the mother country and, at the same time, remarkably isolated.

The Canadian colony offered little to attract immigrants. The fur trade constituted the main economic activity. The overwhelming presence and influence of the military (which contributed 35 percent of the immigrants) on most aspects of colonial development reflected the fact that New France was, at least in the eyes of its masters, little more than a strategic outpost from which to do battle with France's perennial rival, Great Britain.[24]

After an initial period during which New France in effect was run by a royal fur-trading company, the One Hundred Associates, and considerable authority rested with missionary orders, especially the Jesuits, the government of Louis XIV established direct control over colonial affairs. In 1663, the office of intendant for New France was established in Quebec. Appointed by the Crown and responsible for all civil government—justice, finance, and police, which included health matters—the intendant reported directly to the minister of the navy in Paris. Military and foreign affairs in New France remained under the responsibility of the governor general, who also reported to the minister of the navy. In 1674, the Crown named the first bishop of Quebec. Thus the civil, military, and religious administration of New France became tightly incorporated in principle and, to a large extent, in practice into the centralized framework of the French absolute state. Other aspects of social organization in New France, such as the seigneurial system of land tenure and the *coûtume de Paris* (a body of legislation dealing with common law, weights and measures, and the regulation of guilds) were transplants from the mother country. Few of the leading officials in New France were Canadian-born, and most viewed their posts only as career waystations before returning to France. Colonial culture, having no indigenous newspapers or other publications, remained tightly controlled by the French state and church.

The Pattern of Diseases

The diseases afflicting the inhabitants of New France were basically the same as those in France, since most epidemics in the colony literally arrived on ships from the mother country. The religious nursing sisters of the Hôtel-Dieu of Quebec, themselves originally transplants from the mother house at Dieppe, recorded the arrival of the king's vessels each year with a mixture of joy and anxiety because these ships bearing vital supplies also filled their hospital to overflowing with cases of "malignant fevers" such as typhus, typhoid, and influenza. The first epidemic of smallpox (1640) to ravage the Indian population came shortly after the arrival of the nuns at Quebec. Often, pestilences were identified simply by the name of the infected ship, for example, the epidemic of the *Rubis* in 1740 and that of the *Léopard* in 1756.[25]

The pattern and impact of epidemics in New France reflected the peculiar conditions of the colony. Thus smallpox never settled into the endemic childhood pattern characteristic of eighteenth-century French cities. Four major smallpox epidemics struck the colony: in 1640, 1702–1703, 1732–33, and 1755–57. The nursing sisters estimated that the outbreak in the early years of the eighteenth century claimed the lives of one-fourth of the population. This was doubtless a gross exaggeration, but the parish registers indicate a mortality of perhaps as much as 5 to 10 percent of the inhabitants.[26] With wide intervals between epidemics, a considerable proportion of the adult population lacked immunity conferred by previous exposure. New France, like the mother country, did not implement systematic smallpox inoculation; the first such effort came only after the British conquest.

The prevalence of scurvy, a vitamin deficiency disease characterized by generalized weakness and bleeding of the gums, bore witness to the harsh conditions and short supplies of fresh fruits and vegetables in New France. From Cartier's initial encounter with the disease (and his well-known description of the probably efficacious Indian remedy of a beer-like potion derived from the bark and needles of a conifer) until the end of the French regime, scurvy remained a major killer, especially during periods of famine associated with wartime blockades. It was the most common ailment among the troops at Louisbourg on Ile-Royale (Cape Breton Island). Despite Cartier's testimony on behalf of the Indian cure, French medical authorities, like the army physician Chardon de Courcelles, who came from Brittany to Halifax in 1745, remained skeptical of its efficacy after repeated clinical failures. More than 600 persons died from scurvy during the final winter of the French possession of the town of Quebec (1759–60).[27]

New France evidently was spared the bubonic plague. Alerted by the epidemic at Marseilles, the intendant and the governor general imposed a quarantine on the port of Quebec from 1721 until 1724. The only ship to arrive from Marseilles was given a clean bill of health.[28] On the other hand, the colony suffered a serious outbreak of yellow fever in 1710–11, a malady rare in France. Intermittent fever or malaria, a significant problem in many parts of France, seems not to have been so in Quebec, though it was present in the French settlements around the Great Lakes and, of course, in Louisiana.[29]

The cold and damp climate favored a profusion of upper respiratory ailments, lung diseases, and rheumatism among the native Indian population as well as the French settlers. In the winter of 1700–1701, an epidemic—probably influenza—struck Quebec. Its symptoms consisted of a "bad cold" complicated by fever, rib pain, rapid dissemination from person to person, and high mortality.[30] Among endemic diseases, pneumonia and tuberculosis claimed a heavy toll. A sample of death notices of the nursing sisters of the Hôtel-Dieu of Quebec showed nearly 30 percent died from chest diseases.[31] Pehr Kalm, a Swede who visited New France in 1749, reported the prevalence of pleurisy, tapeworm, and venereal diseases.[32] The last-named ailments typically posed a major problem, given the large forces of soldiers and sailors in the colony.

Kalm subscribed to the widely held notion that Europe produced healthier inhabitants than the New World. The French, he believed, lived longer than their Canadian counterparts, who degenerated with each succeeding generation.[33] The notion of New World degeneration did not appear to rest on any empirical evidence. New France, as we have seen, experienced a steady natural increase in population due to a very high birth rate. On the other hand, mortality rates matched those of the mother country. In one striking instance, a leading surgeon of Quebec who sired a grand total of twenty-four children saw all but five die before reaching adulthood.[34] The countervailing myth to degeneration, that the New World retained traces of a disease-free "golden age" supposedly enjoyed prior to contact with the white man, certainly no longer held for the seventeenth and eighteenth centuries.

Organization of Medical Practice

In principle, the organization of medical practice in New France followed closely the pattern of the mother country. To say that barriers between physicians, surgeons, and apothecaries broke down would be to misconstrue the situation. There were in fact almost no practitioners with medical degrees in the colony; only one medical doctor, Jean-François Gaultier (1708–1756), immigrated, and another, Michel Sarrazin (1659–1734), settled in New France as a surgeon before subsequently completing medical studies at Rheims and returning to the colony as a physician. Despite the absence of any organized body of medical doctors, much less a French-style medical faculty, these few physicians, along with several others upon whom the title physician (*médecin*) was conferred by the government, enjoyed higher status and prestige than surgeons in New France.

The office of "king's physician" at Quebec eventually came to be the leading medical post in the colony. Appointed by the minister of the navy, the royal physician did not necessarily hold a university medical degree. His duties, for which he received an annual stipend, included the post of physician at the Hôtel-Dieu of Quebec, the treatment of soldiers, sailors, and the poor, and the expectation that he would contribute to knowledge of the flora and fauna of the colony. As the ranking medical authority in New France, the king's physician at Quebec presided over meetings of his colleagues, the surveillance of apothecaries, and the examination of prospective surgeons.[35]

Surgeons were the ordinary practitioners of medicine in New France just as they were in the mother country, particularly in remote areas of the kingdom. Thus, of some fifty medical men who appear in the *Dictionary of Canadian Biography* for the period of the French regime, all, except the few cited above, were surgeons, a pattern typical of the French organization of medicine whether in the diocese of Auch-en-Gascogne in the mother country or Quebec in the New World.

It is not possible to say with precision how many "surgeons," that is, practitioners of medicine, lived in New France at any given time or even during the entire period of French rule. Like practitioners in the mother country, and perhaps to an even greater extent, many simply set up in practice with healing but one pursuit among a mixture of various other occupations. No clear demarcation separated the regular surgical profession from less well-established "charlatans." Thus a certain Marguerite Dizy, residing at Bastiscan, Quebec, signed a medical certificate in 1730 describing a beating and wounding in which she identified herself as a "chirurgienne."[36]

Surgeons arrived with the earliest colonists. Between 1629 and 1633, no fewer than twenty-two surgeons or apothecaries appear in archival records.[37] Each ship departing France on a long voyage was required to have at least one surgeon or barber-surgeon aboard. In addition, army units came well equipped with medical men. In 1665, for example, Vincent Basset du Tertre arrived in New France as surgeon major with the Carignan-Salières regiment. He was accompanied by twenty-four *fraters* or army barber-surgeons, some of whom remained in the colony when the regiment disbanded.[38] Similarly, during the war of conquest (1755–1760), nearly eighty *fraters* came over with the troops.[39] From the *DCB* sample, it appears that about 80 percent of the surgeons of New France were born in the mother country, and of that group, 80 percent entered the colony as army surgeons or ship's surgeons.

It seems clear that New France had an abundance of surgeons. Using data from 1663, Marcel Trudel counts seventeen members of the "health professions" for a staggering proportion of nearly six practitioners per 1,000 inhabitants. At the beginning of the eighteenth century, the proportion remained equally impressive — nearly 100 surgeons for a population of about 15,000. According to E.-Z. Massicotte, at least seventy-seven such "professionals" settled in the Montreal region during the French regime; the town of Montreal had five in 1669, when there were only a few hundred inhabitants. A prominent Quebec surgeon requested in 1712 that the maximum number of master surgeons in the town be limited to four "without, however, prejudicing those already practicing who shall be permitted to continue until their death or departure from town."[40]

Such high proportions of surgeons in the population would defy belief were it not for factors already mentioned. First, one must remember that the military presence in the colony meant a large supply of medical personnel. Second, the dispersion of the population over a very large, often impassable, territory gave smaller settlements a strong incentive to cultivate and rely on local practitioners. In dealing with small numbers, even a single practitioner results in a deceptively high medical density. Jacques Dugay (1647–1727), for example, practiced for more than fifty years at Trois-Rivières, for a long time as the only surgeon.[41] But, since Trois-Rivières had only a few hundred inhabitants, Dugay by himself gave the town a high medical density.

Third, and perhaps most pertinent, standards for medical practitioners tended to be even more permissive or more difficult to enforce in New France than in rural France. It seems likely that the bulk of ordinary practitioners or surgeons were at best semi-skilled, occasional healers, who practiced with minimal training and no formal examination or licensing. Gabriel Nadeau lists eleven barbers and wigmakers in the town of Quebec in 1742, most of whom, like Pierre Le Breton, *dit* la Lancette, practiced some surgery.[42] Even in Paris, combining the occupations of surgeon and barber was not formally prohibited until 1743, although the majority of master surgeons had long ceased this practice.

Medical practice in New France, however, was not completely open and unregulated. Medical men developed professional structures, albeit rudimentary ones, derived from those in the mother country. Still, well-organized surgical communities or guilds did not appear in the towns of New France. This was probably due to the three factors mentioned above, which reduced the incentive for practitioners to seek to become legitimate master surgeons. But a lieutenant of the king's premier surgeon served at Quebec as the titular leader of the surgeons, barbers, and wigmakers of New France, just as surgical lieutenants presided over their colleagues in hundreds of other towns in provincial France. A surgical lieutenant purchased his office from the premier surgeon at Versailles, and his duties, as the latter's representative, included presiding over the examination and licensing of surgeons and the inspection of instruments and drugs.[43]

Sketchy evidence suggests that the lieutenant at Quebec carried out identical functions. The first holder of this office, Jean Madry (?1625–1669) acquired his post from the king's premier barber in France in 1658. Madry was succeeded first, it seems, by Jean Demosny (1643–1687), and then by Gervais Baudoin (?1645–1700), who served as lieutenant under premier surgeon Charles-François Félix until his death. In 1709 Jourdain Lajus became surgical lieutenant to Georges Mareschal, a post he retained under Mareschal's successor, François La Peyronie, until his own death in 1742.[44]

Little is known about the tenures of the earlier lieutenants, but Baudoin and Lajus, it appears, fulfilled their functions and enjoyed the benefits of office. Lajus presented the petition of 1712 seeking to protect the surgeons of Quebec from competition by outsiders, especially ships' surgeons. On behalf of his fellow surgeons, Lajus brought suits against several "charlatans" or illegal practitioners, and he presided over the licensing of surgeons. In return, Lajus was exempted from several taxes and from service in the militia. After his death, the post of surgical lieutenant apparently lapsed as the king's physician assumed the leading role in professional regulation. An ordinance promulgated by the intendant François Bigot in 1750 declared that all surgeons would be required to undergo a "serious examination" given by the royal physician at Quebec, but candidates for the Montreal and Trois-Rivières regions continued to be examined by the king's surgeon.[45]

Since the majority of surgeons of New France were born in France, they typically trained in the mother country or en route to the colony. Among those mentioned in the DCB as being natives of New France, at least five apprenticed under their fathers.[46]

Several apprenticeship contracts show that this institution was transmitted more or less intact from the mother country. These documents, prepared by notaries, were the means by which a master surgeon and the apprentice (or his family acting in his behalf) settled on the terms of service for a specified period, normally two to three years, as was the custom in France. In 1715 and 1717, Simon Soupiran the elder (1670–1724), master surgeon at Quebec, signed two apprenticeship contracts in which he promised to instruct young men (one age fifteen, the other perhaps slightly older) and to provide food, lodging, and specified supplies or services — in one case, two pairs of French shoes; in the second, laundry, razors, and surgical instruments.[47] Soupiran, who held a hospital post, agreed to let his apprentices visit the hospital when they were not otherwise employed in his service. In return, the young men agreed to do barber's work in Soupiran's shop and various domestic chores. Soupiran apparently had a flourishing business as a barber, including a scheme whereby customers, for a fee of ten *livres*, could purchase a year's worth of shaves and beard-trimming.[48] The apprentices did this work, while the masters, like many of their counterparts in eighteenth-century France, increasingly limited their activities to surgery. Monetary payment to the master surgeon is not explicitly mentioned in these contracts, as it normally was in French apprenticeship arrangements. One Quebec contract — between Jean Demosny and the family of Ignace Pellerin, dated 1676 — mentions, however, the considerable sum of 200 *livres*.[49]

If apprenticeship practices in the colony conformed to those in France, subsequent phases of training remained ill-defined. Little is known about regulations for journeymen surgeons in the colony, and, except for sons of masters, one cannot trace any careers from apprentice through to master surgeon. In the absence of guilds (and thus of serial archives, which one finds for French provincial communities), perhaps no strict rules applied to post-apprenticeship training. It is likely that even more practitioners than in France never bothered to stand for examination or acquire licenses. One rare reference to a journeyman in fact concerns a court decision in his favor, permitting him to leave the service of a master and requiring the latter to pay 25 *livres* for three months' service. (Journeymen were paid by their masters in France as well but had to serve for three years to qualify for provincial guilds.)

The journeyman in question, René Gaschet (?1665–1744), did practice surgery for a time but later became a notary.[50]

Formal public courses in medicine did not exist in New France. Nor, with the exception of a few well-established master surgeons like Madry and Sarrazin, did practitioners return to France for further study. (A return to France, of course, was often a one-way trip during the French period and, even more so, on the eve of and after the conquest.) An intriguing reference to a "school" for young surgeons in Montreal is associated with the name of Jean Martinet de Fonblanche (1645–1701), a surgeon at the local Hôtel-Dieu. Martinet's school for surgical apprentices enrolled two students in 1674 and others as late as 1691.[51] This was perhaps an instance of private initiative by a leading surgeon to take students on a fee-paying basis, a variant of the normal apprenticeship and not an unusual practice in France. Nothing is known of the content of Martinet's teaching at Montreal, or whether this institution survived his death.

Midwives in New France tended to be older married women or widows. Unlike surgeons, few midwives had salaried posts, and most were natives of the colony or long-term residents. In 1721 a licensed midwife of Paris was sent to Louisiana, and the following year Madelaine Bouchette, age thirty-nine, went to Quebec as midwife at a stipend of 400 *livres* per year.[52] Surgeons evidently did not have as much jurisdiction over midwives as they did in the mother country, but they were expected to instruct the women and to aid them in difficult deliveries. Midwives were elected by the married women of each parish, a practice not generally followed in the mother country, where men selected midwives in most provinces. There were, however, precedents in the northeast of France for women to choose their own midwives.[53] In both mother country and colony, midwives took oaths of office from the parish priest in which they promised to follow good Catholic precepts such as refraining from baptising infants except in dire emergencies or from doing anything to endanger the life of the fetus. The royal government launched an effort to improve midwivery, and specifically to train younger, better-educated women, but this occurred in the latter eighteenth century after the loss of the New World colony.[54]

Secular apothecaries were rare in New France. The town of Quebec did not list a single apothecary in a census in the early

1740s. As in smaller French provincial centers, surgeons took over this trade; at Quebec, masters like Lajus, Soupiran, and the Arnoux brothers ordered drugs from France and maintained well-stocked shops.[55]

The religious orders in New France, especially the Jesuits, carried on a tradition of practicing pharmacy among the native Indians and colonists. One Jesuit, Brother Jean-Jard Boispineau, even served as consultant apothecary to the Hôtel-Dieu of Quebec in 1730s and 1740s and taught his brother, also a Jesuit, the apothecary's craft.[56] Many of the hospital nursing sisters acquired competence in the preparation and use of medicinals. The Reverend Mother Marie Catherine Tibièrge de Saint Joachim, for example, earned praise in her death notice as "a long-time *apothicairesse*, . . . a skillful *pharmacienne* consulted confidently by many sick persons."[57] The mother superior and chronicler of the Hôtel-Dieu, Marie-Andrée Duplessis de Sainte Hélène, conducted a regular correspondence with apothecaries in France for some four decades (1718–58). In particular, Mother Sainte Hélène ordered medical supplies from an apothecary at Dieppe.[58] The Hôtel-Dieu also imported drugs from Paris, Bordeaux, and La Rochelle and devoted about one-half of its budget to the purchase of remedies. Pharmaceutical supplies also reached New France via army stocks and by the direct distribution of remedy boxes to parish priests.[59]

The hospitals of New France reflected their counterparts in France. Founded by the royal government or by wealthy benefactors ultimately related to the Crown, such as the Duchesse D'Aguillon, niece of Cardinal Richelieu, who endowed the Hôtel-Dieu of Quebec in 1639, the hospitals depended on the Crown for funds and on nursing orders of the Catholic church for their day-to-day operation. Following the typology of hospitals in the mother country, the Hôtels-Dieu (founded in Quebec in 1639, Montreal in 1643, and Trois-Rivières in 1694) treated medical and surgical patients, while the Hôpitaux-Généraux (Montreal in 1688 and Quebec in 1692) received the old, infirm, mentally ill, and some criminals.[60] Sometimes, however, these distinctions between hospitals broke down, as, for example, during an epidemic when the Hôpital-Général would also receive the acutely ill. At Louisbourg on Ile-Royale, a well-equipped 100-bed Charité hospital (founded 1722) run by monks of Saint-Jean-de Dieu extended

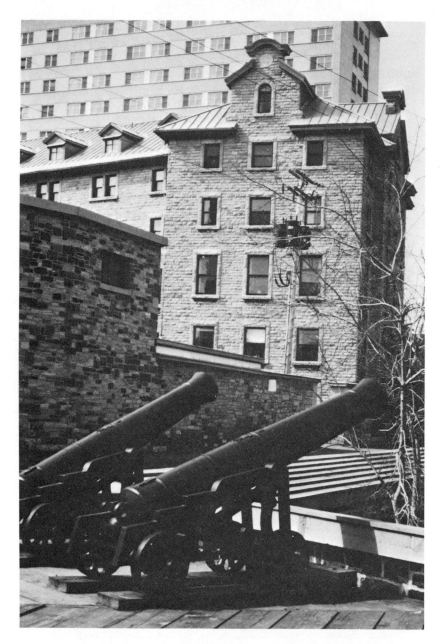

A modern photograph of the Hôtel-Dieu of Quebec City from the ramparts of the Old City. On the original site are hospital buildings constructed between 1850 and 1969 and adjacent to monastery buildings dating from the end of the seventeenth century. Courtesy of Toby Gelfand.

the network of similar hospitals in France and her Caribbean colonies.[61]

The religious sisters received high praise for their hospital service from military and civilian authorities, as well as from travelers in New France. André Doreil, financial commissary of wars at Quebec from 1755 to 1758, extolled the sisters' merits, at the same time urging them to serve wine to patients so that hospital care in New France would match that of the mother country in every detail.[62] Pehr Kalm observed that the Hôtel-Dieu of Quebec was a model of cleanliness, with curtains on the beds, separate rooms for the severely ill, and daily visits by an attending physician and surgeon.[63]

The hospitals of New France compared favorably with the best institutions in the mother country. This is perhaps because they were, in principle, military establishments in which injured and ill soldiers and sailors had priority over civilian patients. Nonetheless, as François Rousseau has demonstrated in a quantitative study of the Hôtel-Dieu of Quebec for the period 1689 to 1698, military personnel constituted little more than one-fifth of some 5,000 admissions during this relatively tranquil decade.[64]

Rousseau argues persuasively that the Hôtel-Dieu at the end of the seventeenth century was well integrated into Quebec society and performed a vital function for the entire population of the surrounding region. Its fifty beds enabled Quebec to match the hospital bed-per-population ratio of the best-endowed provinces in France.[65] As many as 5 percent of the settlers had recourse to the Hôtel-Dieu during the decade, although native Indians, for whom the institution was originally envisaged, no longer constituted a large group of admissions. In contrast to the mother country, even well-to-do persons availed themselves of the hospital: "it is customary in this country for everybody to let themselves be taken there when sick—the powerful, the rich, and all the clergy—and this is because there is easy access to the doctor and to appropriate remedies and because of the special attention given to patients by the nursing sisters."[66]

Nearly twice as many men as women used the Hôtel-Dieu. Male admissions peaked during the spring and summer months, a period corresponding to the activities of farming, navigation, and military maneuvers. This suggests, in the absence of any description of diseases in the records, that the hospital in fact treated

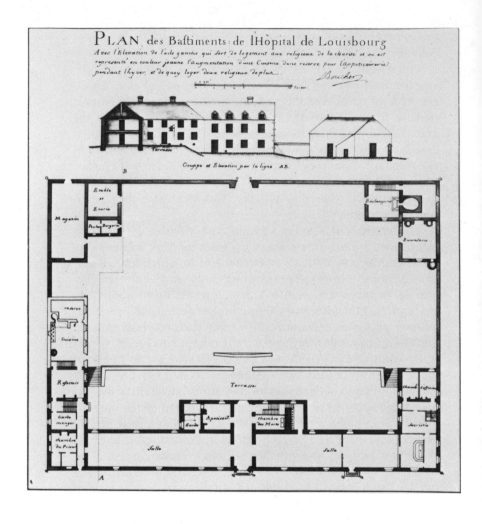

Plan of the charity hospital at Louisbourg on Ile-Royale (now Cape Breton Island), founded in 1722. Courtesy of the Archives Nationales du Canada, Colonies (C11 C16, 1st partie, no. 38).

acute medical conditions, rather than serving simply as a shelter. Women were not admitted for childbirth, nor were infants or young children generally received at the Hôtel-Dieu. As one would expect, mortality rates in hospital exceeded those for the population as a whole. But, with mortality only slightly over 7 percent on the average (deaths could rise dramatically to as high as 25 percent of admissions during epidemics) the Hôtel-Dieu of Quebec did not have the dreaded reputation of the Hôtel-Dieu of Paris, where over 20 percent perished. On the other hand, certain French provincial hospitals had equally low mortality rates. All in all, the several hospitals of New France, well endowed, well administered, and well served by religious and medical personnel, represented an implantation in the New World of a progressive type of French enlightenment institution.

As in small, remote towns of the mother country, local inhabitants entered into contracts with practitioners to ensure their medical care. Thus in 1655 the surgeon Etienne Bouchard signed an agreement to tend all the medical needs of forty-six Montreal families, "except for the plague, the great pox, leprosy, the *mal caduc* [epilepsy], and the operation for the stone." In exchange, Bouchard received a subscription fee of 100 *sous* annually from each family.[67] Evidently, the same surgeon had in 1653, prior to his departure from France, signed another contract in which he promised to serve in Montreal for five years in return for his lodging, nourishment, surgical instruments, an annual stipend of 150 *livres*, and his return passage at the end of the period. The second contract apparently superseded the first, perhaps when Bouchard decided to stay in the colony. Several Montreal practitioners, including Bouchard, signed agreements to work together, entering into partnerships that pooled patients, instruments, and other resources.[68]

Hospitals also contracted for the services of medical men. In 1681, the Hôtel-Dieu of Montreal employed two surgeons for the sum of 75 *livres* per year to attend the hospital on a daily basis, each serving in rotation for three-month periods.[69] At Quebec, a long series of "king's physicians," beginning with Robert Giffard in 1640, served the local Hôtel-Dieu.[70] A goodly number of salaried public medical posts, many related to the military or the clergy, helped New France attract and maintain competent medical men. In this respect, Quebec and Montreal doubtless offered more opportunities than towns of comparable size in France. Simon Soupiran the younger (1704-1764), for example, held posts as surgeon to the admiralty of Quebec, surgeon to the Ursuline convent, and medical "expert" for the lower courts. In addition, and in some measure as a consequence, Soupiran had a large private medical practice.[71]

Jean-François Gaultier received a yearly stipend of 800 *livres* as king's physician in 1741 when ordinary worker's wages were about one *livre* per day.[72] His predecessor, Sarrazin, had received only 600 *livres* per year despite his frequent complaints about his salary. Gaultier also obtained special bonuses during two years plus appointments as physician to the Hôtel-Dieu and to the seminary of Quebec. Finally, he acquired a lucrative fur-trading concession as well as fishing rights off the Labrador coast and an appointment as an assessor on the Conseil Superieur, the highest court in New France.

Another successful surgeon, Robert Giffard (1587–1668), one of the earliest practitioners in New France, became a vigorous colonizer, landowner, and, as seigneur de Beaufort, one of the first recipients of letters of nobility in the colony.[73] Charles Feltz (1710–1776) carved out a highly successful and varied career as a Montreal surgeon. As surgeon-major of the town, he earned 1008 *livres* per year and another 300 *livres* for tending to the Indians. Marriage into a leading fur-trading family gave Feltz entrée into the best society. Eventually, he acquired several homes, speculated in land and medical remedies, and owned ten slaves.[74] Other practitioners combined surgery with other pursuits or turned to new careers altogether. The *DCB* mentions "surgeons" who became successful as fur traders, landholders, brewers, millers, farmers, shipbuilders, notaries, and judges.

It is possible that prospects for upward mobility for surgeons were better in New France than in the mother country. In any case, the hope of improving one's economic and social standing along with the pursuit of a military career and, in some cases, religious convictions must have provided the main incentives for surgeons or would-be surgeons to make the journey to the colony. If they served for six years (a term later extended to ten years), they had the right to be received as master surgeons anywhere in France, including Paris.[75]

Medical Theory and Practice

Given the absence of organized medical faculties or even any physicians from Paris or Montpellier in New France, one is tempted to speculate that European medical theories did not penetrate the colony. Cartier's remark that the Indian remedy for scurvy "has had such an effect that if all the physicians of Louvain and Montpellier had been present with all the drugs of Alexandria, they would not have been able to do in one year that which this tree [the white pine] has accomplished in six days" seems to support the proposed contrast between New World empiricism and Old World tradition.[76]

At any rate, it seems plausible that contact with new remedies loosened the hold of traditional medical thought. Remarks by other travelers in New France raise the same possibility. Louis Antoine de Bougainville noted that Indian healers in general were as effective as European physicians, despite an entirely different set of remedies; the Indians had little use for bloodletting and no knowledge of chemical remedies.[77] Pehr Kalm observed that the Indians did not use mercury to treat venereal diseases, as did Europeans, but achieved good results with roots unknown to the French.[78]

Certainly, native remedies intrigued and even won over some colonists in New France as well as interested parties in the mother country. French apothecaries requested ginseng root, "beaver kidneys" (musk glands), various gums, maple sugar, and other medicinals from Canadian correspondents, and they were willing to trade European remedies for these exotic substances.[79] Sarrazin and Gaultier, both accomplished naturalists and correspondents of the Paris Academy of Sciences, sought to uncover the medical virtues of new plant and animal species they had found.[80]

Thuya wood found use as a salve for rheumatism as well as for coughs and intermittent fevers. Leaves of the herb known as "maiden hair" assuaged consumption, cough, and other chest ailments. An enema of tobacco smoke reportedly could resuscitate a drowned person.[81] The Jesuit surgeon François Gendron (1618–1688) concocted an ointment for treating ulcers and cancers from powdered stones he found on the shores of Lake Erie; on his return to France, Gendron acquired fame with this remedy, which he used to treat Anne of Austria's breast cancer in 1664.[82]

Yet it would be illusory to suppose that these new remedies brought about any fundamental change in medical theory. Most, if they did not already fit in with existing theory (and sometimes with practice), could easily be integrated into the framework of traditional thinking. New mineral springs reported by Kalm would simply be added to the long list of healing waters in France. Rave notices on turpentine derived from the bark of balsam fir trees —"a marvelous remedy for all wounds"— had ample precedent in the surgical literature. The action of a plant root as a cure for epilepsy was explained in terms of its promoting sweating, vomiting, and purging.[83] The remedy might be new, but the medical theory was as old as the Hippocratic notion of restoring a proper humoral balance by evacuation.

The medical practice of a Sarrazin involved frequent recourse to bloodletting, purging, and other traditional modes of therapy followed in the mother country. To the extent that one can evaluate the practice of other medical men in New France from fee bills, lists of drugs ordered and prescribed, and a few court cases, phlebotomy retained its place as a sovereign remedy.[84] Michel Bertier (1695-1740), king's surgeon at the Hôtel-Dieu of Quebec, was accused of hastening a bishop's death with "all too frequent bloodlettings."[85]

Surgery in New France evidently could not rival that in the major centers of the mother country. Operations such as cutting for stones of the urinary bladder and for repairing anal fistulae were performed on occasion, but such procedures were not done on a regular basis in the colony, as they were in French cities. Sarrazin, the most skillful surgeon in New France, however, did amputate limbs and remove cancers of the breast. In at least one instance, he certified that miracle healing at the shrine of Sainte-Anne-de-Beaupré had succeeded in healing a crippling wound where secular medicine had failed.[86] Another surgeon, Henri Lamarre, *dit* Bélisle, had the same experience with a patient whose severed tendon of the leg he could not reunite.[87]

CONCLUSION

As in so many other domains, New France imported its medical knowledge and practices along with its personnel, institu-

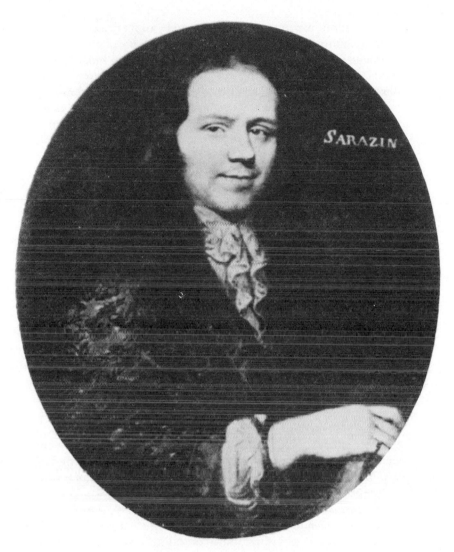

Portrait of Michel Sarrazin (1659-1734). Courtesy of Reverende Soeur Claire Gagnon, a.m.j., archiviste, Les Augustines de la Miséricorde de Jésus Monastère de l'Hôtel-Dieu de Québec.

tions, surgical instruments, and even many of its drugs from the mother country. The rich holdings of the library of the College of Jesuits in Quebec included many medical works. Indeed, with some 130 titles, medicine held a place second only to religion in the library.[88] These books, all of French provenance and mostly published in the seventeenth and eighteenth centuries, tended on the whole to arrive in New France within a remarkably short time after publication. Although the typical practitioner did not have access to this kind of library, the few books that he consulted were likewise of French origin.

We have seen that medical organizations in New France remained close to their Old World origins. The similarities are striking when one compares surgical structures in New France with their counterparts in the provinces of the mother country. In certain areas—for example, the apprenticeship and the office of lieutenant of the premier surgeon—little changed in the passage to New France. As in the mother country, surgeons and barber-surgeons, some licensed as masters and probably more unlicensed, constituted a remarkably numerous collection of ordinary practitioners.

In other respects, the pattern of medical organization underwent some modification in the colonial setting. Formal guilds did not develop. In consequence, the qualifications for practice remained poorly defined despite regulations for examinations. Surgeons did not exercise the same jurisdiction over midwives that they did in France. There were no schools offering public medical courses, as there were in many provincial centers of late eighteenth-century France. The virtual absence of physicians removed opportunities for corporate rivalries and conflicts, common in eighteenth-century France. On the other hand, the few physicians in the colony enjoyed an undisputed professional authority that would have been envied by their French counterparts. Hospitals in New France were well-established medical institutions serving the entire community. In addition to providing medical care, hospitals, along with several other urban institutions in the colony, provided public posts for medical men.

Many of the above variations in the medical structure of New France can be traced to the military and religious presence in the colony, factors that remained more pervasive, or at least more concentrated, there than in the mother country. It must always be borne in mind that French rule terminated abruptly just one decade into the second half of the eighteenth century, at a time when medical change and professional reform were accelerating in France. One can only speculate how much the stunted professional picture in the colony (and its slight development under British rule) might have changed under French "enlightenment." Some medical men departed with the conquest, although many more remained and took an active part in medical affairs alongside their new British colleagues. On the one hand, it seems probable the conquest of 1760 retarded the development of the medical profession and its institutions in French Canada, where a medical society and school did not emerge until the 1820s and then under British auspices. On the other hand, New France's demographic and economic situation, which made it of marginal interest to its French masters, helped precipitate the loss of the colony, and these factors probably would not have changed greatly under continuing French rule.

NOTES

Research for this paper was supported by a grant from the Hannah Institute for the History of Medicine (Toronto, Canada). I acknowledge with thanks the research assistance of Mary Antonnette Flumian, graduate student, Department of History, University of Ottawa. I also wish to thank Laurent Messier and Jacques Bernier.

1. Pierre Goubert, *L'Ancien Régime I: La Société* (Paris: Armand Colin, 1969), *passim*, esp. 31–50.

2. Jean-Pierre Peter, "Disease and the Sick at the End of the Eighteenth Century," in *Biology of Man in History*, ed. Robert Forster and Orest Ranum (Baltimore: Johns Hopkins Univ. Press, 1975), 95–100, esp. 97. See also Fernand Braudel, *Civilisation Materielle et Capitalisme* (XV-XVIIIᵉ siècle) (Paris: Armand Colin, 1967), I:58–68, esp. 59–60.

3. Peter, "Disease and the Sick," 113–24; J. Rousset, "Essai de pathologie urbaine: les causes de morbidité et de mortalité à Lyon aux XVIIᵉ et XVIIIᵉ siècles," *Cahier d'Histoire* (1963), 8:71–105. For rural areas, see the excellent regional monographs by François Lebrun, *Les Hommes et la Mort en Anjou aux XVIIᵉ et XVIIIᵉ Siècles* (Paris: Mouton, 1971); and Jean-Pierre Goubert, *Malades et Médecins en Bretagne 1770–1790* (Paris: Klincksieck, 1974).

4. Peter "Disease and the Sick," 115–16.

5. Ibid., 116–18.

6. Rousset, "Essai de pathologie urbaine."

7. Ibid.

8. Paul Delaunay, *La Vie Médicale aux XVIe, XVIIe et XVIIIe Siè-cles* (Paris: Hippocrate, 1935); Toby Gelfand, *Professionalizing Modern Medicine: Paris Surgeons and Medical Science and Institutions in the 18th Century* (Westport, Conn.: Greenwood Press, 1980), *passim*, esp. 28–30, 41–43.

9. For supporting references to the preceding paragraph and what follows, see ibid. and Toby Gelfand, "The Decline of the Ordinary Practitioner and the Rise of a Modern Medical Profession" in *Doctors, Patients, and Society: Power and Authority in Medical Care*, ed. Martin Staum and Donald Larsen (Waterloo, Ontario: Wilfrid Laurier Univ. Press, 1981), 105–29.

10. Toby Gelfand, "Medical Professionals and Charlatans: The Comité de Salubrité enquête of 1790–91," *Histoire Sociale-Social History* (1978), 11:62–97.

11. Ibid.

12. Muriel Joerger, "The Structure of the Hospital System in France in the Ancien Régime," in *Medicine and Society in France*, ed. Robert Forster and Orest Ranum, trans. Elborg Forster and Patricia Ranum, (Baltimore: Johns Hopkins Univ. Press, 1980), 104–36.

13. Shelby T. McCloy, *Government Assistance in Eighteenth-Century France* (Durham, N.C.: Duke Univ. Press, 1946), 169–70.

14. Jean Verdier, *La Jurisprudence de la Médecine en France* (Alencon, 1763), 2:14–22; Gelfand, "Medical Professionals and Charlatans," 69–70.

15. Caroline Hannaway, "The Société Royale de Médecine and epidemics in the Ancien Régime," *Bulletin of the History of Medicine* (1972), 47:256–73.

16. Shelby T. McCloy, *Government Assistance during the Plague of 1720–22 in Southeastern France* (Durham, N.C., Duke Univ. Press, 1938); Louis LaFond, *La Dynastie des Helvétius: Les Remèdes du Roi* (Paris: Occitania, 1926).

17. Owsei Temkin, *Galenism: Rise and Decline of a Medical Philosophy* (Ithaca, N.Y.: Cornell Univ. Press, 1973), 135–36, 156–58; Howard M. Soloman, *Public Welfare, Science, and Propaganda in Seventeenth-Century France: The Innovations of Théophraste Renaudot* (Princeton, N.J.: Princeton Univ. Press, 1972), 162–200; William Coleman, "Health and Hygiene in the Encyclopédie: A Medical Doctrine for the Bourgeoisie," *Journal of the History of Medicine* (1974), 29:399–421.

18. Martin Staum, *Cabanis: Enlightenment and Medical Philosophy*

in the French Revolution (Princeton, N.J.: Princeton Univ. Press, 1980), 78–93.

19. Peter, "Disease and the Sick"; Hannaway, "The Société Royale de Médecine."

20. François Quesnay, *Essai Physique sur l'économie animale* (Paris, 1747), I:lx–lxvii.

21. Genevieve Miller, *The Adoption of Inoculation for Smallpox in England and France* (Philadelphia: Univ. of Pennsylvania Press, 1957).

22. Erwin H. Ackerknecht, *Therapeutics from the Primitives to the 20th Century* (New York: Hafner, 1973), 65–92; Gelfand, *Professionalizing Modern Medicine*, 9.

23. For general background on New France, see Marcel Trudel, *Initiation à la Nouvelle-France* (Montreal: Holt, Rinehart et Winston, 1968); Marcel Trudel, *La population du Canada en 1663* (Montreal: Fides, 1973); Guy Frégault, *Canadian Society in the French Regime*, The Canadian Historical Association Booklets, No. 3 (Ottawa, 1971). In this paper, the term "New France" refers to the Canadian colony. Unless mentioned specifically, other French possessions in the New World (Acadia, Louisiana, the Great Lakes and Mississippi settlements) are not included.

24. W.J. Eccles, "The social, economic and political significance of the military establishment in New France," *Canadian Historical Review* (1971), 52:1–22.

25. Pierre-Georges Roy, "Les épidémies à Québec," *Bulletin des Recherches Historiques* (hereafter cited as *BRH*) (1943), 49:204–12.

26. Ibid., 207–208.

27. Jean Des Cilleuls, "L'Oeuvre du service de santé au cours de la guerre de 1755–1760," *Histoire de la Médecine* (May 1960), 10:19; Archives historiques de la guerre (Vincennes, France), A' 3417, 128, 310; P. Keisser, "Etude historique sur Chardon de Courcelles," *Bulletin de la Société Académique de Brest* (1900–1901), 26:240–43. There has been some confusion about the identity of the tree used to treat scurvy; see Virgil J. Vogel, *American Indian Medicine* (Norman: Univ. of Oklahoma Press, 1970), 84–86.

28. P.-G. Roy, "La quarantaine sous le régime français," in *Les Petits Choses de Notre Histoire* (Québec: Lévis, 1919), 1:129–32.

29. Pehr Kalm, *Peter Kalm's Travels in North America, The America of 1750*, ed. Adolf B. Berson (New York: Dover, 1966), 370.

30. P.-G. Roy, "L'épidémie de grippe de 1700–1701," *BRH* (1921), 35:547–48.

31. François Rousseau, *L'Hospitalisation en Nouvelle France: l'Hôtel-Dieu de Québec, 1689–1698* (Quebec: Université Laval, 1974), thèse de maîtrise.

32. Kalm, *Travels*, 370, 499.

33. Ibid., 499.

34. Peter N. Moogk, "Jourdain Lajus," in *Dictionary of Canadian Biography* (hereafter cited as *DCB*) (Toronto: Univ. of Toronto Press, 1974), 3:344–45. All references to the *DCB* are to the English edition. Vols. 1 and 2 appeared in 1966, vol. 4 in 1979. The French version of this bilingual project is published by Laval University.

35. Gabriel Nadeau, "Le dernier chirurgien du roi à Quebec, Antoine Briault, 1742–1760," *L'Union Médicale du Canada* (1951), 80:705–26, esp. p. 709.

36. "Un Compte de 'Chirurgienne,'" *BRH* (1926), 32:167; Raymond Douville, "Chirurgiens, barbiers-chirurgiens et charlatans de la région trifluvienne sous le régime français," *Cahiers des Dix* (1950), 15:81–128.

37. Joseph-Edmond Roy, *Histoire du Notariat au Canada,* 4 vols. (Québec: Lévis, 1899–1902), 1:8–10.

38. G. Nadeau, "Vincent Basset du Tertre," in *DCB*, 1:79–80.

39. Nadeau, "Le dernier chirurgien du roi," 721.

40. Trudel, *La population du Canada en 1663,* 100–102; Mary Loretto Gies, *Mère Duplessis de Sainte-Hélène, annaliste et epistolière* (thèse de doctorat) (Québec: Université Laval, 1949), 119; E.-Z. Massicotte, "Les chirurgiens, médecins . . . de Montréal sous le régime français," *Rapport de l'Archiviste de la Province de Québec* (hereafter cited as *RAPQ*) (1922–23), 3:131; Sylvio Leblond, "La législation médicale à la période française," in *Trois Siècles de Médecine Québeçoise* (Quebec: La Société Historique de Québec, 1970), 27. The request to limit the number of practitioners was rejected.

41. Raymond Douville, "Jacques Dugay," *DCB*, 2:202–203.

42. Nadeau, "Le dernier chirurgien du roi," 719–20.

43. Ibid., 714–15; J.-E. Roy, *Histoire du Notariat,* 12–14.

44. See articles on "Madry," "Demosny," "Gervais Baudoin," and "Jordain Lajus" in *DCB*.

45. *BRH* (1913), 19:339–41.

46. Jean Demosny the younger, Gervais Baudoin the younger, Antoine-Bertrand Forestier, François-Xavier Lajus, Simon Soupiran the younger. See respective articles in *DCB*.

47. "Un engagement d'apprenti chirurgien en 1717," *BRH* (1926), 32:541; "Chirurgien et barbier," *BRH* (1942), 48:285; Robert-Lionel Séguin, "L'apprentissage de la chirurgie en Nouvelle France," *Revue d'Histoire de l'Amérique Française* (1967), 20:593–99.

48. Peter N. Moogk, "Simon Soupiran," *DCB*, 2:613–14.

49. M.-J. and G. Ahern, *Notes pour servir à l'histoire de la médecine dans le Bas-Canada* (Quebec, 1923), 139–41.

50. Michel Paquin, "René Gaschet," *DCB*, 3:236–37.

51. Charles-Marie Boissonnault, "Jean Martinet de Fonblanche," *DCB*, 2:465–66.

52. Nadeau, "Le dernier chirurgien du roi," 723–25.

53. Jacques Gélis, "Sage-femmes et accoucheurs: l'obstétrique populaire aux XVIIe et XVIIIe siècles," *Annales: Economies, Sociétés, Civilsations* (1977), 32:927–57, esp. 934–36.

54. Ibid., 938–51.

55. Nadeau, "Le dernier chirurgien du roi," 723.

56. Ibid., 722; Antonio Drolet, "Florent Bonnemère," *DCB*, 1: 107–08; M. Giovanni, "The Role of the Religious in Pharmacy under Canada's 'Ancien Régime,'" *Culture* (1963), 24:13–32.

57. Annales de l'Hôtel-Dieu de Québec de 1755 à 1774, fol. 18, in Archives de l'Hôtel-Dieu de Québec.

58. M.L. Gies, *Mère Duplessis de Sainte-Hélène, passim*; Nova Francia (1929), 4:368–80; (1930), 5:359–79.

59. Nadeau, "Le dernier chirurgien du roi," 721–22.

60. Among numerous monographic studies, see Jeanne-Françoise Juchereau de Saint-Ignace et Marie-André Duplessis de Sainte Hélène, *Les Annales de l'Hôtel-Dieu de Québec, 1636–1716* (Montreal, 1939); Micheline D'Allaire, *L'Hôpital-Général de Québec, 1692–1794* (Montreal: Coll. Fleur de Lys, 1971); Marie Morin, *Annales de l'Hôtel-Dieu de Montréal* (Montreal: Impr. des Editeurs, 1921); Maria Mondoux, *L'Hôtel-Dieu, premier hôpital de Montréal, 1642–1763* (Montreal, 1942).

61. Hermas Bastien, *L'Ordre hospitalier de St-Jean-de-Dieu au Canada* (Montreal: Lumen, 1948).

62. "Lettres de Dorcil," *RAPQ* (1944–45), 25:66–67.

63. Kalm, *Travels*, 446. See also Nicolas-Gaspard Boucault, "Etat présent du Canada (1754)," *RAPQ* (1920–21), 1:40–41.

64. François Rousseau, "Hôpital et Société en Nouvelle France: L'Hôtel-Dieu de Québec à la fin du XVIIe siècle," *Revue d'Histoire d'Amérique Française* (1977), 31:29–47, esp. 34–45. The following three paragraphs are based upon this source.

65. Ibid., 46. For France, see Jeorger, "The Structure of the Hospital System in France," 117–18.

66. Dom Georges-François Poulet, "Récit simple de ce qu'un réligieux bénédictin a souffert au Canada au sujet de la bulle Unigenitus," cited in Rousseau, "Hôpital et Société," 42.

67. Massicotte, "Les chirurgiens, médecins . . . de Montréal," 132, 146.

68. J.-E. Roy, *Histoire du Notariat*, 15–16.

69. Massicotte, "Les chirurgiens, médecins . . . de Montréal," 149–50.

70. M.L. Gies, *Mère Duplessis de Sainte-Hélène*, appendice C.

71. Moogk, "Soupiran," *DCB*, 3:595–96.

72. Bernard Boivin, "Jean-François Gaultier," *DCB*, 3:675–78.

73. Honorius Provost, "Robert Giffard de Moncel," *DCB*, 1:330–31.

74. Gilles Janson, "Charles Feltz," *DCB*, 4:264–66.

75. Nadeau, "Le dernier chirurgien du roi," 716–17.

76. Quoted in Des Cilleuls, "L'Oeuvre de service de santé," 19.

77. Bougainville, "Le Mémoire sur l'Etat de Nouvelle France (1758–59)," *RAPQ* (1923–24), 4:69–70. Indians did, however, practice phlebotomy.

78. Kalm, *Travels*, 390. In his report to the Swedish Academy, Kalm identified the root as lobelia. According to Bougainville, the Indians' remedies for venereal diseases were "tisanes composées de quelques simples," which achieved "paliative" rather than "curative" results.

79. Antonio Drolet, "Quelques remèdes indigènes à travers la correspondance de Mère Sainte-Hélène," in *Trois siècles de médecine Québecoise*, 30–37.

80. Boivin, "Gaultier," *DCB*, 3:675–78; Arthur Vallée, *Un biologiste canadien, Michel Sarrazin, 1659–1735: Sa vie, ses travaux et son temps* (Québec: Imprimerie du roi, 1927), 81–128.

81. Kalm, *Travels*, 438, 469; N. de Dièreville, *Relation of the Voyage to Port Royal in Acadia or New France (1699–1700)*, ed. John C. Webster (Toronto: Champlain Society, 1933), 180.

82. G. Nadeau, "François Gendron," *DCB*, 1:328.

83. Kalm, *Travels*, 471, 491; Dièreville, *Relation of the Voyage to Port Royal*, 176–77, 181–82.

84. Vallée, *Un biologiste canadien*, 57–60; Massicotte, "Les Chirurgiens, mèdecins . . . de Montréal," 151–54; "Un plaidoyer pour services médicaux en 1759," *BRH* (1930), 36:634–40.

85. C.-M. Boissonnault, "Michel Bertier", *DCB*, 2:60.

86. Vallée, *Un biologiste canadien*, 60–65, 251–54.

87. P.N. Moogk, "Henri Lamarre," *DCB*, 2:339–40.

88. Antonio Drolet, "La Bibliothéque du Collège des Jésuits," *Revue d'Histoire d'Amérique Française* (1960–61), 14:487–502.

3

Medicine in New England

ERIC H. CHRISTIANSON

In 1734 Dr. John Perkins of Boston visited London to "see what they had in practice new, or better than we had." Despite finding vast environmental differences between the teeming English metropolis and his provincial hometown, he concluded that medical practice was much the same in both places. Other, more recent, observers have argued that the distinctive conditions of New England substantially altered the medical institutions and practices of the Old World.[1] In this essay, based on a survey of existing literature, I have sought to adjudicate between these two views by examining the medical history of colonial New England, particularly that of Massachusetts, against the background of developments in Old England.

ENGLAND

At the time of Queen Elizabeth's death in 1603, England did not possess a profitable and well-organized colonial empire like Spain's.[2] With some Crown control, enterprising individuals and joint-stock companies, rather than the English monarchy itself, colonized and exploited the new lands. The conditions of life in England combined with the prospects of living in new lands to attract thousands of eager settlers for these endeavors. The individualism of the optimist and of the opportunist provided the momentum for English expansion.

Between 1600 and 1700 the population of England and Wales increased from about four million to over six million. By the end of the eighteenth century the number of inhabitants had grown to over nine million, with London accounting for about 10 percent of the total.[3] Although the vast majority lived in communities of less than 5,000 inhabitants, a few provincial towns in 1700 — Norwich, York, Bristol, Newcastle, and Exeter — boasted populations of between 10,000 and 20,000.[4] From the southwest and southeast came the largest flow of early immigrants to the North American colonies, organized by ambitious businessmen and God-fearing reformers seeking a diversified labor force to support their overseas ventures.[5] Included in the cultural baggage of these immigrants to the New World were their experiences with disease, their medical practices, and their medical organizations.

Diseases

Any attempt to classify the diseases of the seventeenth and eighteenth centuries involves hazards for the historian because diagnosis was often imprecise. As one medical historian has noted, it is difficult, if not impossible, even to distinguish between such diseases as diphtheria and scarlet fever "when eighteenth century doctors themselves made no attempt to separate them."[6] Nevertheless, contemporary records and epidemiological patterns reveal much about the medical problems of Stuart and Georgian England. Perhaps the most familiar medical event is the epidemic of bubonic plague that took over 60,000 lives in London in 1665.[7] But the English also suffered from smallpox, syphilis (also called the great pox or French pox), measles, malaria, dysentery (the bloody flux), pneumonia, tuberculosis (consumption), dropsy (congestive heart failure), and stones in the urinary bladder. The last condition was so prevalent in England during the eighteenth century that one observer speculated that enough bladder stones could be found to "macadamize [pave] one side of Lincoln's Inn Fields."[8] Some diseases, such as smallpox, became endemic and distinguishable from others with somewhat similar symptoms, such as measles; beginning in 1629, London's Bills of Mortality separated the two diseases.[9] By 1700, smallpox had become the most common mortal disease of English childhood, with the possible exception of infantile diarrhea.

Such figures are based on the experience of London, where there were more record-keeping practitioners, governmental agencies, and medical institutions than in the countryside. We do not possess enough evidence at this time to tell if life in the larger provincial towns was more conducive to longevity than life in London. The belief of some contemporaries, however, that living in rural areas favored healthier, if not longer, lives has received qualified endorsement from recent scholars who have proposed that "inhabitants in smaller towns in both America and Europe had greater life expectancies than did those in larger communities."[10]

Medical Practitioners

A variety of healers provided medical care in England: physicians, surgeons, apothecaries, and other ordinary practitioners, as well as ministers, midwives, nurses, grocers, traveling mountebanks, and patients themselves, who bought over-the-counter medicines from chemists or concocted home-made simples.[11] The dominant medical institutions in London were the three corporations that separated members from ordinary practitioners and protected the interests of physicians, apothecaries, and surgeons.

During the first half of the sixteenth century, King Henry VIII granted charters to the Royal College of Physicians of London (1518) and to the United Company of Barber-Surgeons of London (1540), thus giving them independence and autonomy. Apothecaries won similar concessions from King James I in 1617, when he bestowed corporate privileges on the Guild of Apothecaries of London, separating them from grocers. These institutions created a medical hierarchy with physicians on top. As one early seventeenth-century observer put it, the physician was the "great commander [who] has subordinates to him, the Cooks for diet, the Surgeons for manual operation, and the Apothecaries for confecting and preparing medicines."[12] By the opening decades of the seventeenth century, which coincided with the initial phase of English colonization in North America, the essential institutional structure of the London medical community was in place.

This tripartite division of functions, however, could not be maintained strictly by these corporations. Although not necessarily without training or experience, unlicensed practitioners flourished in London, and they were dominant in the provinces.[13] In theory the medical corporations and guilds protected London physicians, surgeons, and apothecaries from would-be competitors in other guilds and from nonmembers in the provinces. According to medical statutes, physicians were to limit their practice to diagnosis, prognosis, and prescription. Apothecaries were to prepare medications prescribed by physicians. The activities of surgeons were limited to extracting teeth, letting blood (phlebotomy), treating skin lesions, and performing such operations as amputations and lithotomies for the removal of stones in the urinary bladder—all of which they could do either on their own or at the direction of a physician. But in 1745, King George II granted surgeons their own London guild, thus depriving barbersurgeons of the right to perform lucrative major operations and to consult with physicians.[14] Although charged with maintaining the boundaries between specialties, the corporations for a number of reasons were unable to do so. Among the destabilizing factors were increased educational opportunities, the ambition of apothecaries and surgeons to usurp the functions of the more prestigious physicians, and the growth of the medical marketplace.

Many barber-surgeons, surgeons, apothecaries, and ordinary practitioners ignored the medical statutes and continued to practice medicine along with surgery or pharmacy. Attempting to guard its regulatory power over this diverse group of healers in London, between 1581 and 1600 the Royal College of Physicians prosecuted at least 236 individuals for practicing medicine without a license.[15] In response to their critics' derisive claim that they were uneducated pretenders (the physician was to be a university medical graduate), apothecaries established in 1627 a seven-year apprenticeship for those hoping to join the ranks. Pointing with pride to their lengthy and supervised period of training, they defended their increasingly physician-like functions. After all, they argued, who knew more than they about the substances, both botanical and chemical, from which prescriptions were prepared and about the actions of these prescriptions on patients. The appearance of standardized pharmacopoeias in English would eventually assist the apothecaries in their quest to expand their role.

So, too, did the great London plague in 1665, during which many physicians retreated to the safety of the countryside, leaving ordinary practitioners, including apothecaries, surgeons, and barber-surgeons with most of the responsibility of caring for the sick.[16]

The frequent and bold intrusions of apothecaries into the domain of physicians prompted the College of Physicians to seek legal redress. In the celebrated Rose Case of 1703, pitting an apothecary practicing medicine against the college, the House of Lords granted apothecaries within the jurisdiction of London permission to function as ordinary practitioners of medicine.[17] As apothecaries practiced more medicine and surgery, druggists, or chemists, increasingly took over the preparation and sale of drugs.

During the first half of the eighteenth century, London's physicians continued to express much concern over the blurring of corporate distinctions. Increased educational opportunities, over which the college exercised little direct control, facilitated the upward mobility of the lower ranks. The medical, surgical, and midwifery personnel at the hospitals and medical schools of Leiden and Paris continued to attract English students well into the eighteenth century.[18] But the founding of new hospitals in London, such as Guy's, Middlesex, and the Westminster Lying-In, convinced many others to study at home. These hospitals allowed their staff medical personnel to offer instruction and demonstration to private pupils.[19] The availability of this training certainly benefited the surgical specialist and male midwife, both of whom were more likely to reside in larger communities, as well as the apothecary-surgeon. As the dominant type of practitioner in the provinces, apothecary-surgeons practiced medicine, prescribed the drugs that they prepared, and usually limited their surgical intervention to minor operations.[20]

As formal instruction became increasingly important for these medical practitioners, many traveled north to Scotland to obtain an M.D. degree from one of the new medical faculties at Edinburgh, Aberdeen, or St. Andrews. These schools did not admit female practitioners, but did accept male dissenters from the Church of England who would not have been admitted to the universities at Cambridge and Oxford. The Scottish schools offered both beginning medical students and veteran apothecary-surgeons, at least the men, a relatively quick way to join the ranks of the physician by obtaining degrees. During its early years the Royal

College of Physicians had granted licenses to those who had se-
cured the endorsement of a respected physician and had passed
an examination to determine competency, but by 1750 the academic M.D. degree had become virtually the only acceptable
qualification for practicing medicine in London.[21] The college responded to these changing educational opportunities for would-
be physicians by attempting to prevent degree-holding apothecary-
surgeons, who lacked training in the liberal arts, from practicing
in London. Presumably more interested in practicing than in being prosecuted, apothecary-surgeons who earned Scottish M.D.'s
settled, or relocated, in the villages and towns of the provinces.
Some returned to care for their former patients and sought to increase the size and diversity of their clientele in areas where the
regulatory powers of the college were weak.

Although the terms "physician" and "doctor of medicine" had
always been synonymous, many who called themselves "doctors"
did not restrict themselves to diagnosis or prescription. By the
second half of the eighteenth century this situation led some physicians in London, and even in the larger provincial towns, to call
for a new name more "descriptive of the physician's circumstances," a replacement for this "antiquated and prostituted title."[22]

Even before the creation of London's medical corporations, a
statute enacted in 1511 established a basis for organizing and
regulating medical practice throughout provincial England.[23] This
law placed the licensing of physicians, surgeons, and other practitioners under the church. In 1643, parliament abolished the ec-
clesiastical hierarchy, thus suspending episcopal licensing until it
was re-instituted in 1660. Licensing under this arrangement proved
to be inconsistent, and the level of the bishop's attentiveness in
this matter varied considerably throughout the realm. University
licenses were not covered by the 1511 statute and remained valid
except in London. In effect, access to practice the healing arts was
open to all under common law; licensing remained a route to
legitimation rather than a means to seek permission to practice
as a physician, surgeon, or other practitioner. The right, not the
competence to practice, was the issue here. Over time, academic
credentials made the distinctions between the titles of physician,
surgeon, or apothecary less confusing, but they did not eliminate the controversy over appropriate medical functions.[24]

Studies of the differences, as well as of the similarities, between the organization of medical practice in London and in the provinces have become methodologically refined. Several studies based on fragmentary data have offered approximations of the number of practitioners and their ratios to population in selected locations and periods of time. A conclusion shared by these studies is that the number of practitioners throughout England has been vastly underestimated. The results of some analyses also suggest that differences between the organization and practice of medicine in London and in the provinces have been overestimated. Although admittedly incomplete, these data permit some illumination of the differences and similarities. The research focuses largely on the period 1580–1643, during the latter part of which New England was settled, with much less available for the late eighteenth century, when the colonies declared their independence.

For the period 1580–1643, recent studies have been concerned with communities in East Anglia, a major supplier of immigrants to New England. Located in the counties of Norfolk and Suffolk, the most thoroughly studied towns are Norwich, King's Lynn, and Ipswich. With a population of about 17,000 in 1600, Norwich was the second largest city in England. At least seventy-three people have been identified as practitioners in Norwich for 1580–1600.[25] Quite similar in its diversity to other provincial towns, the listing of Norwich practitioners has been reported as: 37 surgeons or barber-surgeons, 12 apothecaries, 10 women practitioners, 6 practitioners of physic, 5 academically trained physicians, and 3 miscellaneous practitioners. Comparable to findings for King's Lynn and Ipswich, a Norwich practitioner "might hold a license in medicine or surgery or both from the University of Cambridge, the Bishop of Norwich, the Archbishop of Canterbury or a variety of agencies in London, including the Bishop of London and the Privy Council."[26] These communities also served as temporary residences for itinerant practitioners who moved about the countryside.[27] Ordinary practitioners, especially surgeons and barber-surgeons, and not physicians, were the largest numerical group in East Anglia.[28] Much the same can be said of London where in 1600 only fifty of its estimated 500 practitioners were physicians.[29] From results obtained from limited data, it would seem that physicians generally constituted less than 20 percent of the medical practitioners in any community. This diversity, if not also the dominance of the ordinary practitioner, has been implicitly suggested by a study of a later period.

Between the accession of King James I in 1603 and the temporary abolition of episcopal licensing in 1643, a date coinciding with the end of the Great Migration to New England, one study reports the presence of 814 men licensed to practice medicine in "the villages and hamlets of provincial England."[30] Of this total, the vast majority (604 or 74.2 percent) had attended college, and 76 percent of this number had received a bachelor's degree. Although nearly one-third (250 or 30.7 percent) possessed an M.D. degree, better than one out of five (22 percent) neither attended college nor received any documentable formal training. While it demonstrates the minority status of physicians, two critics of this study conclude that it does not take into account a much larger group of healers, such as those identified in Norwich. For East Anglia, it is "doubtful whether even freemen, or licentiates, represent a majority of those dispensing medical care.[31]

A crude approximation of the ratio of practitioners to population is possible for the period 1580–1643. In Norwich, Ipswich, and London, the ratios of practitioners to population around 1600 have been estimated at 1:220–250, 1:208, and 1:400, respectively.[32] The evidence remains too sketchy to make the claim that smaller communities generally had more practitioners than did larger ones. Future analyses of practitioners not consistently included in available studies (such as women practitioners, midwives, and nurses) would, however, undoubtedly yield higher ratios of practitioners to population in all communities than have been reported in the literature. Lacking analyses of numerical data for the eighteenth century, long-term comparisons are not possible at the present time.

Perhaps because of the diversity of practitioners, most of whom were also engaged in other income-producing activities, provincial towns seem to have been less rigid in organizing and regulating medical practice. With membership open to all categories of practitioners, medical societies in the provinces during the eighteenth century reflected a spirit of cooperation among members that did not exist between London's corporations. In contrast to the Royal College of Physicians of London, preoccupied as it was well into the eighteenth century with regulating practice, the corporations for apothecaries and surgeons took an active role in the training of their apprentices and the continuing education of their members. London's three royally chartered corporations differed markedly in composition, though not always in all functions, from medical societies created in London and in the provinces.

Between 1757 and 1836 there were many medical societies in London, some of them quite short-lived.[33] A few, such as the Society for the Improvement of Medical and Chirurgical Knowledge (1783), catered to the needs of specific medical corporations, yet disregarded their functional distinctions. Three of the societies active during 1795–1815 were rather inclusive in composition within the context of the teaching hospital.

Hospitals like Guy's, Middlesex, and St. Bartholomew's attracted physicians, surgeons, apothecaries, and pupils who enrolled under their supervision to study medicine and its various branches. Advances in knowledge and skill brought them closer together in spite of their separate corporate or noncorporate origins. Records of these societies remain fragmentary. For the Guy's Hospital Physical Society, founded in 1771, the breakdown of each category by percentage of the total membership in 1804 of 659, less six clergymen, was 13 percent M.D.s, 20 percent surgeons, less than 1 percent apothecaries, and 65 percent (431), who "had no professional identification and probably were surgeons, apothecaries, or practicing as both."[34]

Quite similar to contemporary philosophical and natural history societies, mutual interests brought diverse groups together in Guy's Hospital Physical Society. Its members were "desirous of improvements in Medicine, and the other Sciences nearly allied to it, and convinced of the numerous and great Advantages, arising from a free communication of Observations and Opinions."[35] Not all of the members were general practitioners, but they expressed the "general practitioner's interest in, and understanding of, both medical and surgical problems."[36] Provincial societies, open to all established medical practitioners, surgeons, apothecaries, and their apprentices, also stressed the importance of appreciating the complementary nature of the various branches of medicine.

In 1774, Robert Richardson Newell, an apothecary-surgeon practicing in Colchester, East Anglia, organized the first of the provincial societies.[37] Newell's father, also an apothecary-surgeon, practiced in nearby Harwich, and his wife's father was an apothecary in Colchester. Newell apparently served an apprenticeship with his father, a practice more common among apothecary-surgeons in the provinces than among physicians in London. The varied membership of this society suggests an absence of fixed professional boundaries; among the six original members besides Newell, there were two M.D.s (Cambridge and Edinburgh), an apprentice-trained apothecary, an apothecary-surgeon, a surgeon, and a surgeon-midwife. Other provincial societies, such as those in Plymouth (1794) and Leicester (1800), also defied the functional distinctions of London's guilds, a practice that certainly reflected the realities of medical practice in rural areas. These societies assisted in the training of apprentices, fostered professional improvement, and helped solve disputes among members. Their appearance outside of London suggests that even in the provinces the need to improve skills and expand knowledge within a formal context was increasing.

Medical Theory and Practice

At the most general level the practice of seventeenth-century physicians differed little from that of physicians in ancient Greece and Rome.[38] In both eras physicians possessed three techniques by which to determine the nature of an illness: listening to the patient's own description of symptoms, observing the patient's appearance and behavior, and examining the patient's body.[39] To these verbal and visual techniques, the eighteenth-century physician added procedures that were increasingly manual, such as performing percussion.

Medical theory and therapeutics in the seventeenth century continued to be strongly influenced by humoralism, formalized by Galen in the second century A.D. Basically, this tradition maintained that health resulted from a natural balance of bodily humours (yellow bile, blood, phlegm, and black bile) and their manifested qualities (cold, heat, moistness, and dryness). When not associated with injury due to physical trauma, disease was thought to result from an imbalance of the humours. To restore balance, physicians administered preparations of natural substances, either topically or internally. Feverish patients, for example, would be advised to follow a cooling regimen; they might also be bled to help eliminate excess heat produced by too much blood. Those suffering from chills and a runny nose would take preparations that warmed and dryed. If a patient's stool was abnormally dark, the physician might conclude that there was an excess of black bile and prescribe an enema or an orally administered laxative. The followers of Galen thus advocated an active role for the physician in the management of disease.

During the seventeenth century continental influences and a renewed interest in Hippocratic doctrines affected both medical theory and practice in England. By 1600, the influence of Paracelsus (1493–1541) was increasing.[40] This revolutionary Swiss physician taught that diseases were real entities produced by specific causes. An advocate of mineral or chemical remedies, he was successful in convincing pharmacopoeia compilers to include mercury (for syphilis), lead, sulphur, iron, arsenic, copper sulfate, and potassium sulfate in the published drug lists. Apothecaries and apothecary-surgeons were certainly in a position to expand their functions by popularizing and taking advantage of this advice.

The most important seventeenth-century proponent of Hippocratic teaching was Dr. Thomas Sydenham (1624–1689), who based his medical practice, and instruction, on an eclectic combination of ancient and modern theories.[41] As an admirer of Hippocrates and believer in the healing power of nature, the *vis medicatrix naturae*, he believed that nature and experience, not theory, should be the healer's guide; this philosophy earned him the title of "The English Hippocrates." His English physician contemporaries often ignored his advice, but colonial American practitioners at least paid him considerable lip service. With the availability of such advice from an Englishman, the physician's competitors were encouraged to broaden the level of their intervention in the management of illness or injury.

In spite of anatomical and physiological attacks on the underpinnings of humoralism during the sixteenth and seventeenth centuries, Galenic doctrines, or some variation of them, found acceptance well into the nineteenth century. But as Galen's authority came to be questioned on many points, various theories were proposed to replace it. Something a diversity of healers had encouraged since antiquity, a by-product of this competition for orthodoxy in medical theory seems to have been a willingness to innovate, to deviate from recommended therapy. For example, in a diary entry for 1602–1603, the writer records how Dr. Henry

Gellibrand of provincial Kent expressed the uncertainties implicit in the therapy that he gave to "a minister, [who] was very sick. Gellibrand gave him a glyster [enema], and let him blood the same day, for a fever; his reason was, that not to let him blood had been very dangerous but to let him blood is doubtful, it may do good as well as harm."[42]

Although medical thought tended toward uniformity in both rural and urban areas, similarities in practice may have been offset by variations in degree. Given the information we now have, we cannot be certain that rural medical practice was less heroic in its use of bleeding and purging than that found in the large towns and cities.[43]

NEW ENGLAND

The North American mainland colonies were the foremost locations for English settlement, followed, not far behind, by Ireland.[44] The period of actual settlement spanned more than a century: from Virginia in 1607 to Georgia in the 1730s. With few exceptions the basic problems of settlement were quickly overcome, and the inhabitants rapidly increased their numbers. From a few thousand sprinkled along 1,000 miles of coastline in 1630, the population grew to 250,000 by 1700; and at the beginning of the American War for Independence in 1776, some two and one-half million people resided there, nearly one-third the number of residents in England and Wales. Not until the time of the first U.S. Census in 1790, did about 3.3 percent of the population live in communities with 8,000 or more inhabitants.[45] To be sure, there were cities in America that surpassed or rivaled the provincial centers in England, the three largest being Philadelphia (42,000 in 1790), New York (21,000), and Boston (18,000). Yet, in 1730, Boston, with 13,000 inhabitants, had led Philadelphia and New York, which each had about 8,500. Throughout the colonial period, New England attracted the most homogenous group of immigrants, who emigrated largely from countries in the west country and East Anglia.

Writing about the growth of New England, which contained about 25 percent of the U.S. population in 1790, is in effect like writing about the expansion of Massachusetts. Under the direc-

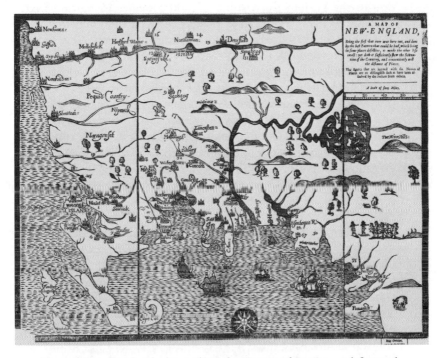

Map of New England, drawn by John Foster of Boston and first published in William Hubbard, *A Narrative of the Trouble with the Indians in New England* (Boston: John Foster, 1677). This so-called "Wine Hills" map (corrected to "White Hills" in later editions) is thought to be the first map engraved and printed in British America. This photograph, courtesy of the Library of Congress, is from a nineteenth-century copy based on the original.

tion of the Puritan elect, some 20,000 provincial English took part in the Great Migration to Boston between 1630 and 1643.[46] Not represented by a cross section of English society, New England was "levelled" at the start. Most of the immigrants belonged to the socioeconomic group called the "common sort," which included farmers, laborers, artisans, and merchants, as well as a variety of medical personnel, ministers, holders of small political offices, and lawyers. Some of these immigrants had attended a university (mostly Cambridge), but most still acquired their expertise through occupational inheritance or by serving an apprenticeship. As congregational or presbyterian dissenters from the Church of England, they preferred local autonomy with the church and town meeting serving as loci of community action.

The Puritan venture to create a city upon a hill, a Holy Commonwealth, ran into difficulty when more immigrants arrived than could be safely located near the colony's center of power, Boston.[47] Immigrants moved out to the north, south, and west, creating the new colonies of Rhode Island, Connecticut, and New Hampshire.[48] Despite being perhaps the most densely populated region in North America, New England remained overwhelmingly rural, with most of its inhabitants residing in small villages and towns that were often named after provincial English towns (Boston, Cambridge, Ipswich) or counties (Norfolk, Suffolk, Essex). In Massachusetts alone, eighty-one towns existed in 1700, and by 1790 another 172 had been incorporated. Given these circumstances, in many ways Boston was to Massachusetts, or to New England, what Norwich was to Norfolk or East Anglia. During the seventeenth century immigration accounted for most of New England's population growth, but later increases from births became more important. During the eighteenth century, the population of Massachusetts doubled every 37.4 years, about ten years longer than it took in the previous century.[49]

Not many colonial communities have received systematic demographic attention, but we know that in Andover, Massachusetts, life expectancy for male children born during the seventeenth and eighteenth centuries exceeded that of English male babies by more than ten years. The high growth rate of Massachusetts also depended upon the ratio of males to females, early marriages, and the generally youthful age of the initial population. Although usually characterized by the dominance of families, both new and established, New England also attracted thousands of indentured servants, who ranged in age from the late teens to the early thirties. In England, conditions forced the postponement of marriage until the man was about twenty-seven and the woman twenty-five, but in Massachusetts the comparable figures were about twenty-five for men and twenty-two for women.[50] All of these factors help to account for the dramatic growth in population. But we must also consider the role played by disease.

Patterns of Disease

Accompanying immigrants to New England, and awaiting them upon their arrival, were various diseases. Investors and boat operators in search of quick profit and settlement leaders eager to secure needed manpower encouraged overcrowding on vessels during trans-Atlantic crossings, which in the seventeenth century lasted two months or more. Navigational improvements eventually reduced travel time to about six weeks, but the growing number of ships and passengers also increased the possibility of disease transfer, particularly those with epidemic potential in a rapidly expanding and mobile population. Although ship-board diets improved over time, scurvy frequently broke out, and poor dietary practices before, during, and after sailing for America probably lowered resistance to many diseases. Carving out an existence on the frontier also involved risk to life and health. During the eighteenth century, improved dietary habits and housing, as well as changes in the distribution of population, reduced the incidence of some diseases, but improved lifestyles also gave rise to medical problems common among prosperous people in England, particularly gout.

The most important epidemic diseases brought to the colonies were smallpox, diphtheria, scarlet fever, and measles. Yet, intestinal problems and respiratory ailments, such as pneumonia and pulmonary tuberculosis, were undoubtedly the major causes of high mortality. It is difficult, however, to determine the cause of death with accuracy for that period because of the ambiguous manner in which doctors recorded the medical problems of their patients.

While relatively free from the epidemic and endemic attacks of yellow fever, malaria, and typhus that plagued settlements to the south, New England was visited by most of the epidemic diseases of the times.[51] The first encounter with smallpox, imported along with the settlers to John Winthrop's Massachusetts Bay Colony, occurred in Boston during the 1630s. Originating in the British Isles, the West Indies, or in Canada, smallpox epidemics ravaged Massachusetts and most of New England in 1648, 1666, 1677, 1689, 1702, 1721, 1731, 1751, 1764, and in the 1770s. During the celebrated epidemic of 1721, during which inoculation was first practiced in America, over half of Boston's 10,670 inhabitants became infected and over 800 died. Death rates from smallpox seldom reached 14 percent in America, which was much better than the 18 to 40 percent that obtained in England during the period. Helping to reduce the severity of smallpox epidemics were effective quarantine measures, isolation facilities, and controlled inoculation campaigns. Smallpox, like dysentery and typhus, often followed the movements of armies, and the colonists waged many campaigns against the French, the Indians, and, of course, the British during the eighteenth century.

Measles, smallpox, and dysentery struck all age groups; diphtheria and scarlet fever, primarily children. First appearing in Boston in 1657, measles continued to be reported for the duration of the colonial period. Apparently the disease more often proved fatal in America and affected a larger number of adults than in England, where frequent epidemics conferred immunity upon those who survived it in childhood. The most destructive measles epidemic of colonial times, the New England epidemic of 1713, claimed over 100 deaths. Late in the eighteenth century, however, the disease seems to have become endemic; by 1800, it was primarily a disease of childhood.

Contemporaries called diphtheria by many names: cynanche, squinancy, quincy, angina, canker, bladders, rattles, hives, throat ail, and throat distemper. Diphtheria was also frequently confused with scarlet fever, which first appeared on the London Bills of Mortality in 1703, and which arrived in New England the year before. In 1735–36, scarlet fever and diphtheria struck simultaneously (for the former, largely in Boston), resulting in the most destructive epidemic of any childhood disease in American history. Whereas scarlet fever claimed over 100 deaths from the estimated

4,000 persons infected, diphtheria in New Hampshire alone took 1,500 from a population of 20,000.

Increased population density during the eighteenth century may also have added to the number of those without immunities, thereby assuring contagious diseases many victims. The incidence of epidemic diseases no doubt produced a widespread sense of vulnerability, regardless of available therapies and variations in mortality rates. Community leaders, concerned about economic disruption and loss of manpower, consulted with local medical practitioners and worked with them to develop public health policies.[52]

Although both New England and the parent country shared many disease experiences, survival rates in America were usually higher. Thus New England was generally a more healthful place in which to live.

The Origins and Training of Early New England Doctors

As late as 1800, neither in New England nor elsewhere in the new nation did there exist effective measures to regulate medical education and practice.[53] This situation prevailed both because of the duration of the initial period of settlement and because of the develoment of local practices in the physically isolated colonies. Although institutional and legislative responses to unregulated practice differed from place to place, the experience of New England, particularly Massachusetts, is well documented and serves as a useful example of this phenomenon.[54]

Of the nearly 1,600 doctors who practiced medicine in Massachusetts between the founding of Plymouth in 1620 and the election of Thomas Jefferson to the presidency in 1800, fewer than 100 were immigrants.[55] Generally the immigrant practitioners came from Great Britain rather than from continental Europe; at least sixty-eight arrived from the British Isles, compared with fewer than ten each from France, Germany, and the Netherlands. About one quarter of them received some form of documented training prior to their departure for America: four served apprenticeships, four earned M.D.s, eight attended universities, and, during the eighteenth century, thirteen gained experience in the armed services of Britain or France. Regardless of their titles and functions in their homelands, in the colonies, where there were no regulations, they became "doctors" and combined the functions of Old World guilds.

Until the middle of the eighteenth century, there are few recorded objections in New England to this free use of the title "doctor." This practice seems to have originated even before the end of the Great Migration to Massachusetts in the 1640s, which included medical practitioners from both London and the provinces. Of the fifty-four English medical immigrants, at least thirty-four arrived before 1700; most of those from other areas came during the eighteenth century. The experiences of four of the twenty-four Englishmen migrating before 1650 reveal the conditions in which "doctor" became a common title for male medical practitioners.[56]

In the log books of the *Mayflower,* which landed at Plymouth in 1620, we find the name Samuel Fuller. A native of Redenhall, Norfolk, where he was born in 1580, Fuller joined the separatists bound for Leiden, the Netherlands, in 1609. It is believed that he studied some medicine in London and may have served an apprenticeship or attended medical lectures in Leiden, where he worked at least part-time as a silk weaver. The ship's log lists Fuller variously as physician, surgeon, and doctor. After his arrival in New England, he was summoned as "Dr. Fuller" by the leaders of Salem and Boston to go north of Plymouth to assist the diseased inhabitants. His use of phlebotomy to treat scurvy indicates that he did not confine his duties, as a physician, to diagnosing and prescribing. He died of smallpox in 1633.

Another *Mayflower* passenger, the surgeon to the ship's crew, was Giles Heale, who had served an apprenticeship and was licensed to practice by the Barber-Surgeons Company of London, which required trans-oceanic passenger vessels to have surgeons.[57] Although his skills were desperately needed in Plymouth, Heale remained only four months before returning to England.

Giles Firmin and his father, an apothecary from Suffolk County, arrived in Boston in 1632. The younger Firmin had attended Cambridge University and then served an apprenticeship with Dr. John Clark in London. For over a decade he practiced in Boston and nearby Ipswich. Responding to the shortage of experienced practitioners, Firmin presented what was perhaps the first series of medical and anatomical lectures in the colonies. At least one of those attending the lectures served an apprenticeship with him. Firmin's suggestion to provide cadavers for dissection before groups of apprentices and practitioners seems to have gained legislative endorsement after his departure for England in 1644 to become vicar of Shalford in Essex. In 1646, the Massachusetts General Court endorsed a proposal that would allow the body of an executed malefactor to be dissected by such groups.

The only M.D. to arrive before 1650 was Robert Child of Norfleet, Kent, the only one of the 814 English country practitioners mentioned earlier known to have visited Massachusetts. In Boston by 1638, he seems to have been more interested in checking up on his business interests than in practicing medicine because local authorities reproached him for neglecting his calling. The Massachusetts Bay government in Boston expelled him for professing unorthodox religious beliefs. Two years later that same government approved legislation that addressed the need for more skilled practitioners to protect residents from the dangerous advice and therapies of the self-proclaimed doctor.

Enacted in 1649, the law applied to "Chirurgeons, Midwives, Physitians, and others."[58] Its origins are distinguishable in the provincial English background of the immigrants, including medical practitioners. By endorsing the introduction of the apprenticeship system and by seeking an examination for competency to practice administered by local practitioners and laymen, the law reflected the customs and practices of rural England. By encouraging competency in more than one type of practice, it further replicated the functional realities of medical organization and practice in provincial England. The blurring of medical functions already evident in England posed no problem in New England, where the "doctor" became a kind of general practitioner.

Immigrant medical practitioners constitute 31 percent of all seventeenth-century doctors in Massachusetts; in the next century they account for only 3.9 percent. Because of the void created by the absence of men like Heale and Firmin and because the 1649 law proved unenforceable, persons claiming medical skills whatever assumed the title "Doctor." In Massachusetts, between 1700 and 1794, 861 practitioners (62.8 percent of 1,370 identified), styled themselves as "doctors."[59] Following the initial period of immigration and settlement, then, medical practice in New England came to be dominated by native-born doctors, most of whom had received no formal training.

For about half of the colonial period the ratio of doctors to population remained stable.[60] In 1650, with fifty doctors serving a population of some 50,000 in Massachusetts, the ratio was 1:1,000. Fifty years later the ratio remained unchanged. During the eighteenth century, however, the ratio steadily increased to 1:569 in 1750 and to a high of 1:417 in 1780. This was much higher than in the new nation as a whole, estimates for which vary from 1:600 to 1:800.[61] At the time of independence, Massachusetts contained about 10 percent of the population of the United States, but approximately 20 percent of its 3,500 doctors. Over a third of its medical practitioners had served apprenticeships, compared to a tenth for the nation as a whole.[62]

Because medicine was rarely a full-time endeavor in colonial America (or England), doctors, like other settlers, moved out of Boston in search of clientele, land, and security. Just as the influx of immigrants into Boston during the seventeenth century had created a demand for medical skills, so, too, did the migration of settlers into Worcester, Hampshire, and Berkshire counties throughout the eighteenth century. There were few large towns at any time in colonial Massachusetts, and those with fewer than 1,000 residents usually had higher ratios of doctors to population (1:557) than did larger communities (1:950). In both England and New England, then, sparsely populated areas seem to have served as residences, both temporary and long-term, for more healers than large towns, where life expectancy was shorter. Although it is doubtful that variations in medical practice were primarily responsible for the differences in life expectancy between rural and urban areas, some doctors expressed concern that the low level of medical training was threatening the health of Massachusetts' inhabitants.

The educational background of New England doctors was as diverse, if not as intensive, as that of English practitioners. Prospective New England doctors did not need to attend college, enroll in hospital lectures, possess an M.D. degree, or even serve an apprenticeship. A few, however, such as Thomas Bulfinch, Sr., received extensive training.

Upon completing an apprenticeship with Dr. Zabdiel Boylston, a respected Boston physician, surgeon, and apothecary-shop owner, Bulfinch sailed for Europe.[63] During the winter of 1718 he observed and practiced the latest surgical techniques at St. Thomas Hospital in London, where he became the first American pupil of the celebrated William Cheselden. Later, Bulfinch crossed the channel and achieved another American first by studying anatomy and surgery with Jean Louis Petit at the Paris Charité Hospital. Returning in 1721 to his native Boston, where his brother, Adino, owned an apothecary shop, he soon married Judith Coleman, the daughter of a prominent minister. Later their son, Thomas, Jr., also chose a career in medicine.

After graduating from Harvard College in 1746, young Bulfinch served a three-year apprenticeship with his father. Encouraged by his father's success, he went to England in 1754 to round out his medical studies. In London he met the king's personal physician and "walked" the famous teaching hospitals—Middlesex, St. Thomas, and St. Bartholomew. Eventually he traveled to Scotland, where he attended the chemistry lectures of Dr. William Cullen and in 1757 received an M.D. degree from the University of Edinburgh. Bulfinch, Jr. subsequently returned to London, to assume a hospital post as consulting physician, but the death of his father forced him instead to sail home to settle his father's estate and take over his large practice. Eventually he took on pupils and apprentices of his own. Given the absence of effective measures to restrict medical practice in New England, young Bulfinch's extensive training was most atypical.

New England's first medical school, created at Harvard College, did not begin accepting pupils until 1783. Founded in 1636, Harvard sought above all to train ministers but also to keep students at home and to help maintain local autonomy. There was little support for creating professional schools of medicine or law until late in the eighteenth century because skills in both fields had traditionally been acquired through the apprenticeship system. Although medical degrees were available in Philadelphia and New York as early as the 1760s, few Yankees went south—or anywhere else—to study.[64] Only about fifty students from Massachusetts went abroad to study medicine and fewer than twenty of those received M.D.s.[65] Between 1749 and 1800, over 100 Americans earned M.D. degrees at Edinburgh, including forty-nine Virginians, fifteen Pennsylvanians, ten New Yorkers, but only four natives of Massachusetts.[66] One eminent New Englander offered an explanation for this provincial, stay-at-home behavior. Benjamin Waterhouse, who had attended lectures at Edinburgh and taken his M.D. at Leiden (1780), once remarked that Americans need not travel to Europe in order to "treat the disorders of their neighbors."[67] Thus most New Englanders who desired medical training took advantage of local opportunities, particularly apprenticeships.

Used in England until the middle of the eighteenth century, when formal academic training replaced it, apprenticeships remained popular in New England into the nineteenth century. Before 1700, only about 140 men, and an undetermined number of women, practiced medicine in Massachusetts, and only about 20 percent of this number were apprentice-trained, most having no formal training at all. This contrasts with the situation in England, where, between 1603 and 1643, four out of five country practitioners had some formal training. Of the 1,370 doctors practicing in Massachusetts between 1700 and 1794, however, at least 488 or 36.6 percent had served apprenticeships.[68]

Although apothecaries and surgeons in England were required to serve apprenticeships lasting up to seven years, the available evidence for Massachusetts suggests that the average apprenticeship there lasted just over one year, five years being the longest. The following apprenticeship agreement, drawn up in Massachusetts in 1736, may be typical of such documents:

> Articles of Agreement Indented and made . . . Between Zabdiel Boylstone of Boston in the County of Suffolk Practitioner in Physick & Surgery of the one part, and Joseph Lemmon of Charlestown in the County of Middlesex, Esqr. on the other part. . . .
> Imprimis - The said Zabdiel Boylstone Doth Covenant and agree for himself to teach and Instruct the said Joseph Lemmon Junr. in the Arts, Mysterys and Businesses of Physick & Surgery during the term of two years . . . and also to find and provide for him good sufficient and suitable Dyet and lodging during the said two years. . . .
> In Consideration whereof the said Joseph Lemmon for himself his Executors and adminrs. doth hereby Covenant and agree to and with the said Zabdiel Boylstone to pay him two hundred pounds in full Satisfaction for his Sons dyet and lodging and for the Instruction

Apprenticeship agreement from 1760 between John McElRoy and
Dr. William Clark (Dolbeare Ms. Folio, 1760–1766). Courtesy of
the Massachusetts Historical Society.

which the said Boylstone shall give him in the said Mysterys of
Physick and Surgery during the term of two years ending in March
1737. . . . [69]

Occasionally, a student would finish an apprenticeship with one
mentor and then continue his studies under the guidance of another; this is what John Perkins did before he visited London in
1734.[70] Some scholars have suggested that the apprenticeship system weakened during the eighteenth century, but in Massachusetts it grew stronger. During the period 1751 to 1790, 45.5 percent of all doctors starting practice were apprentice-trained, an
increase of 28 percent over the pre-1750 period.[71] Obviously, self-
taught "doctors" were most typical of the period, but their shadow-
like appearance in the historical records prevents our making firm
generalizations about them.

Among the most easily identified of the 1,370 Massachusetts
practitioners during the eighteenth century are the 399 (29.9 percent) who attended college, and especially the 360 of this number
who received a B.A. degree.[72] The collegiate curriculum of the day
offered little that would directly benefit a medical practitioner, and a bachelor's degree was not an essential prerequisite
for the M.D. candidate in either Scotland, Leiden, or America.
Of the Massachusetts doctors who attended college, most (86.1
percent) went to Harvard, with the remainder coming from Yale
(8.6 percent), and from American or European colleges and universities (5.3 percent).

Prior to 1700, less than 20 percent of Massachusetts' doctors
attended a college or university, but during the eighteenth century
collegiate preparation became increasingly common. Between 1701 and 1770, college graduates constitute a per decade
average of 33.9 percent of all those starting to practice in each
period. After 1750, Yale and Harvard graduates increasingly
chose to become doctors or lawyers rather than ministers.

Custom dictated that about three years after receiving his
bachelor's degree a graduate would return to his alma mater to
obtain an M.A. degree by submitting and defending a thesis, classical in style and theoretical in substance. To some proud New
Englanders, the M.A. degree represented the epitome of colonial
education—the final polish for young gentlemen. In reality, the
degree was little more than a formality. The subject of the thesis did

Table 1. Percentage of College Graduates Entering the Professions

	1701–45	1778–92
Harvard		
Medicine	13.4	16.9
Law	5.6	33.3
Divinity	36.0	25.6
Yale		
Medicine	6.8	10.4
Law	6.8	30.9
Divinity	50.0	27.7

Source: Eric H. Christianson, "Individuals in the Healing Arts and the Emergence of a Medical Community in Massachusetts, 1700–1794: A Collective Biography" (unpubl. Ph.D. diss., Univ. of Southern California, 1976), 88–89.

not always indicate a career preference; 257 (64.1 percent) of the Harvard graduates who became doctors received M.A.s, yet only 76 (29.6 percent) elected to defend medical or physiological subjects.[73] Since even an M.A. degree did not prepare one to practice medicine, a number of prospective doctors continued their studies abroad.

In 1700, John Cutler of Boston became the first of at least 50 medical students from Massachusetts to study abroad. Of these travelers thirty-five (70 percent) had attended college, and forty-two (84 percent), including many of the collegians, had served medical apprenticeships. Of the forty-three who went to Britain, thirty-eight spent some time in London, and at least twelve attended lectures at one of the Scottish medical schools. Virtually all the Massachusetts doctors who earned an M.D. degree abroad also studied midwifery, anatomy, and surgery in a Paris or London hospital—either before or after graduating from medical school. That so many studied midwifery and surgery suggests that these New Englanders, like their provincial English and Scottish counterparts, had no intention of practicing medicine in the manner of London physicians.

Before 1700, 22 percent of all Massachusetts doctors came from medical families of two or more generations; during the eighteenth century this percentage dropped to 15.7 percent, which suggests that medicine was attracting new names to the ranks. Yet, throughout the colonial period recruitment from medical families accounted for a substantial number of practitioners.[74] Between 1700 and 1794 nearly 20 percent (271) of all Massachusetts doctors either came from or married into medical families. There were at least 215 two-generation families and 52 of three or more generations. All sons in multigenerational families served apprenticeships, customarily with their fathers, but only one out of four attended college, and even fewer, such as Thomas Bulfinch, Jr., traveled abroad or received an M.D.

The tendency of multigenerational medical families to reside in towns of fewer than 1,000 inhabitants contributed to the high ratio of doctors to population in these small communities. Apparently confident of future business and interested in making money as mentors, many medical fathers trained paying apprentices from outside the family as well as their own sons. For example, Dr. Thomas Bulfinch, Sr., not only trained his son, Thomas, Jr., but Benjamin Stockbridge, Jr., and his son, Charles. Bulfinch, like other mentors, consented to train new doctors, and although the Stockbridges did not live in Boston, he was, nevertheless, producing potential competitors in the medical marketplace.

Some evidence suggests that doctors without family connections in the profession may have resented the dominance of multigenerational medical families in some communities. Virtually all of the medical societies in Massachusetts drew their members from the ranks of the apprentice-trained doctors, especially those who had also graduated from college or had gone to Europe or Britain; but only 25 percent of all eligible medical-family members ever joined a county or state medical society.

As an agency for medical education, the multigenerational medical family seems to have assumed a greater importance in New England than in England, although the evidence is limited. While academic training beyond, or instead of, the apprenticeship first appeared in England, by the second half of the eighteenth century medical society organizers were promoting similar reforms in New England. For in Massachusetts, where only one out of three was even apprentice-trained, the ordinary practitioner dominated.

Medical Organizations

Designed to meet a variety of needs, medical societies were created earlier and in greater numbers in Massachusetts than elsewhere in British America, or even, except for the guilds of London and Edinburgh, in Britain.[75] At least seventeen medical societies were either proposed or created in Massachusetts during the eighteenth century, fourteen appearing after 1750. Their goals ranged from proposing minimum requirements for practice, improving the profession's public image, and facilitating self-improvement, to licensing as the only criterion for practice. Although the longevity of some remains uncertain, the locations of all are known; Suffolk County (Boston) supported six, but the majority arose in the country. In terms of the educational background of their members and their stated objectives, a few of the most important groups—notably the Boston Medical Societies of 1735 and 1780 and the Massachusetts Medical Society—resembled London's guilds, without their functional distinctions. Granted the similarities in both composition and function to the provincial and

Table 2. Medical Societies in Massachusetts, 1721–1794

Date	Name	Purposes
1721–22	Club of Physicians (Boston)	oppose inoculation
1726–35	Physicall Club (Boston)	self-improvement
1735–54	Boston Medical Society	self-improvement; combat scarlet fever
1755	Jepson's Proposal (Boston)	self-improvement after apprenticeship
1765	Association of Doctors (Middlesex County)	self improvement; upgrade public image
1766	Ames' Proposal (Middlesex County)	eliminate competition from quacks
1768	Sociable Club (Middlesex County)	self-improvement; eliminate quacks
1771*	Martimercurian (Middlesex County)	self-improvement
1771*	The Spunkers (Middlesex County)	body snatching
1772*	Club of Generous Undertakers (Middlesex County)	body snatching

Table 2. (*Continued*)

Date	Name	Purposes
1780–	Boston Medical Society	repression of quackery by licensing & membership; proposed mandatory lectures at Harvard
1780	The Confederacy of Physicians (Middlesex County)	self-improvement
1781–	Massachusetts Medical Society	regulation by membership & licensing
1787–	Berkshire County Medical Association	self-improvement; regulation by membership & cooperation
1789–	Middlesex County Medical Association	self-improvement; regulation by membership & cooperation
1791–	Bristol County Medical Society	self-improvement; regulation by membership & cooperation
1794–	Worcester County Medical Association	self-improvement; regulation by membership & cooperation

*denotes Harvard College student societies

Sources: Eric H. Christianson, "'To Check the Growth of Imposters': The Role of Massachusetts Medical Societies in Preserving the Apprenticeship System, 1721–1794" (unpubl. manuscript), and "'The Confederacy of Physicians': An Historical Oversight?" *Journal of the History of Medicine and Allied Sciences* (1977), 32:73-78.

student societies of England, most of New England's medical societies were created in response to local problems or the appearance of other societies in the area rather than as a conscious imitation of organizations in England.

Most of the Massachusetts societies proposed more training for medical practitioners; midwifery regulation was not on their agendas. The first explicit call for training beyond the apprenticeship came from the group organized in 1755 by William Jepson, who had recently completed an apprenticeship with Dr. Silvester Gardiner of Boston.[76] In the by-laws of his society, composed of former apprentices interested in improving their knowledge and skills, Jepson enumerated the "many disadvantages attending a separate way of study." Although he had learned much as an apprentice, he realized that there was more to be learned than an apprenticeship could offer. Sharing books, they would first cover anatomy, then surgery, midwifery, physick, and then "proceed to the Other Sciences." Other medical societies, primarily concerned with limiting medical practice to those who could demonstrate adequate training or who could pass a licensing examination, faced the problem of what to do with the hundreds of men already practicing who had received no training at all.

Boston's epidemics of smallpox in 1721 and scarlet fever in 1735 served as major stimuli for the creation of medical societies. The Club of Physicians (1721), the Physicall Club (1726), and the Boston Medical Society (1735) were all created by Dr. William Douglass, a Scotsman with an M.D. from Utrecht.[77] Douglass possessed the only M.D. in Massachusetts at the time, but he was not the only Boston practitioner with European training. For membership in all three of his groups, he selected only men who had graduated from college, served an apprenticeship, or studied in Europe. The 1721 group, though not primarily interested in regulating general medical practice, did oppose inoculating patients against smallpox without quarantining them. When the epidemic passed, the group disbanded. In 1726, Douglass started the Physicall Club with essentially the same personnel, who met occasionally to discuss medical philosophy and therapeutics. When scarlet fever struck Boston in 1735, those same doctors assisted one another in combatting the epidemic; encouraged by this cooperative effort, Douglass organized the first Boston Medical Society.

In 1738, as president of the society, Douglass proposed that qualified practitioners and innocent patients be protected from "Shoemakers, Weavers and Almanack Makers, with their Virtu ous Consorts, who have laid aside the proper Business of their lives to turn Quacks."[78] He advised the General Assembly to enact legislation "so that No person shall be allowed to practice Physick within the limits of this Province" before passing an examination administered by "such regular, approved and learned Physicians and Surgeons as the Honourable Court shall see [fit] to appoint." His provision to include both physicans and surgeons as examiners of candidates for the practice of "Physick" indicates the blurring in New England of the medical functions associated with the London guilds. In view of the great numbers of self-trained practitioners, Douglass advocated a simple solution: regardless of training, anyone who could pass an examination would be judged competent to practice. His proposal paralleled the provisions of the 1649 Massachusetts law, the 1518 charter of the Royal College of Physicians of London, and the 1511 statute of Henry VIII that regulated provincial English practice. Douglass wanted to vest the regulation of medical practice in the hands of a few examining practitioners. The assembly, however, refused to grant a Boston society jurisdiction over medical practice throughout the province. For the duration of the society's existence (it seems to have fallen apart after Douglass' death in 1752), it functioned essentially as an organization for self-improvement, presenting lectures, dissections, and operations to audiences composed of members, interested apprentices, and laymen. This first Boston Medical Society raised issues that would not be forgotten. Throughout the remainder of the eighteenth century, medical-society leaders continued to explore avenues that might eliminate the self-taught.[79]

Most of the medical societies created between 1765 and 1794 were located outside of Boston. The tactics employed by these groups to combat the increase of untrained doctors differed markedly from those originating in Boston. The three efforts that Dr. Nathaniel Ames, Jr. made to organize a medical society in Middlesex County in the 1760s illustrate one approach to the problem. In language reminiscent of Douglass' earlier observations, Ames wrote of men "having Poor stomachs to return to the stall or plough from whence them came; some of them commence QUACKS and call themselves Doctors."[80] In the spring of 1765, the presence of several self-taught practitioners in the area around Dedham, where he lived, prompted Ames and twenty-three other doctors to form a medical society. A letter signed by "Graph Iatroon" (Greek for "writing of physicians") explained that there had been

> some time on foot a proposal forming medical societies or
> Associations of Doctors . . . for the more speedy improvement of
> our young Physicians . . . to get the Profession upon a more
> respectable footing in the Country by suppressing this Herd of

Empericks who have heaped such intolerable contempt on the
Epithet *Country Practitioner.*[81]

The contents of the letter were "carefully sealed and superscribed
lest a telltale Wife or Child divulge that which must be as secret
as Masonry till some Societies are established." Ames and his
friends thought that it was imperative to avoid "degrading each
other . . . before the patient or people by consulting with untrained men." The discord produced by such actions was "highly
detrimental to the Profession" and provided "great advantage to
the ignorant and designing"; in fact, it was the "chief Root from
whence these very Empiricks spring." Although the existence of
this society remained secret, Ames openly pushed for the regulation of medical practice.

Utilizing his popular Almanack to reach a wider audience,
Ames, together with several colleagues, some of whom had recently returned from studying in Europe, continued the war on
quackery. As founder of the Sociable Club (1768), formed to reduce bickering within the ranks of the trained doctors and to
"keep up the Honor of the Profession of Physick," Ames declared
that

> Titles are marks of honest men and Wise,
> The Fool or Knave that wears a title lies.[82]

He advocated warning trained colleagues and unsuspecting patients of the presence of quacks by publicly identifying them. Little came of this particular campaign, but renewed concern soon
produced a more ambitious effort. In 1768, Ames circulated a
copy of John Morgan's treatise on the need for American medical
schools, published in Philadelphia in 1765, in which he warned
the quack, the "remorseless foe to mankind," to hold "thy exter-
minating hand."[83] Morgan himself had helped to found a medical
school in Philadelphia in 1765, and Ames lamented that Massachusetts had allowed a "neighboring province so far to get the
start of us in the regulation of this noble science, which of all others, most needs the protection of civil authority." To prevent medical
practice from remaining open to "every ignorant drone that assumes
the title of doctor," he submitted a bill to the House of Representatives in 1768 for "regulating the Practice of Physick." At the

time, however, the legislature was preoccupied with Samuel Adams' circular letter opposing the Townsend Duties. This is the last known attempt to regulate the practice of medicine until 1780.

The War for Independence during the late 1770s stimulated many of those who served in the medical corps to reevaluate the need for medical regulation.[84] Among these reformers was John Warren of Boston. While at Harvard College in the early seventies, he started three student societies because the school offered no medical lectures. Even after completing his apprenticeship, Warren, like William Jepson and Nathaniel Ames, retained doubts about the limitations of such training. So did his Boston colleague Williams Smibert (M.D., Edinburgh), who observed that American medicine would never become a science as long as students were "taught to believe compleat [sic] medical knowledge is to be acquired in a few months under the tutelage" of someone who himself had not received training beyond the apprenticeship level.[85]

In 1780, Warren and twelve colleagues formed the second Boston Medical Society, demanding for membership not only a completed apprenticeship or its equivalent, but a medical or bachelor's degree as well. Members of the society believed that the existing apprenticeship could not accommodate the tremendous increase of information about medical discoveries and surgical techniques; that Harvard College would have to assume some responsibility for educating doctors by offering a course of lectures; and that quackery, which the legislature failed to suppress, could only be combatted by exclusive societies. Toward this end, Warren urged patients not to patronize self-taught practitioners.

The following year, Warren's group, now fourteen members strong, attempted to convince the state legislature to incorporate them as the Massachusetts Medical Society. But the legislature, which included many representatives from western counties, where distrust of Boston power ran high, insisted that the society expand its membership to seventy before receiving a charter.[86] So, from the more than 600 doctors in the state, about one-third of whom possessed apprenticeship training or more, the society selected an additional fifty-six members. Although the legislature granted the society the privilege of examining and "licensing" practitioners, it failed to provide an effective means of enforcing the society's standards. According to Warren, this legislation per-

MEDICAL PAPERS,

COMMUNICATED TO THE

MASSACHUSETTS MEDICAL SOCIETY.

TO WHICH ARE SUBJOINED,

EXTRACTS from various AUTHORS, containing fome of the IMPROVEMENTS, which have lately been made, in PHYSIC and SUR-GERY.

Publifhed by the SOCIETY.

NUMBER I.

PRINTED AT *BOSTON*, 𝔐𝔞𝔣𝔣𝔞𝔠𝔥𝔲𝔣𝔢𝔱𝔱𝔰,

BY THOMAS AND ANDREWS.

At *FAUST's* STATUE, No. 45, *Newbury Street.*

MDCCXC.

The Massachusetts Medical Society, chartered by the legislature in 1781, produced its first volume of papers in 1790. Courtesy of the Francis A. Countway Library of Medicine.

mitted the society to enable "the people at large (who might otherwise be incapable of fully discerning the qualification of candidates for practice), to distinguish the persons upon whom they may rely."[87] In other words, the profession had received permission to regulate itself, if it could.

In some ways the efforts of Warren and his Boston colleagues resemble that of Thomas Linacre and his five associates who, in 1518, convinced King Henry VIII to incorporate them as the Royal College of Physicians of London. Yet, the Boston society was much more ambitious; it sought control over the entire state, whereas the London physicians had sought merely to monopolize the practice of medicine in London, not in the provinces. In 1785, acknowledging its unrepresentative membership throughout the state, the Boston-based society invited correspondence with groups that may have already been in existence, and encouraged the formation of affiliated county and district medical societies that would recommend candidates for examination and licensing. Apparently, informal associations of practitioners already existed in some locales, but the first counties to organize societies were Berkshire (1787), Middlesex (1789), Bristol (1791), and Worcester (1794). Given the delayed response time (two to nine years) to the 1785 communication issued by the Massachusetts Medical Society, it seems unlikely that county medical society members perceived that their right to practice was threatened legally by the existence of the Boston-based group. They may, however, have sought to protect themselves from competition presented by other practitioners in their communities.

The by-laws of these local voluntary associations indicate a willingness to include any practitioner who wished to improve himself and his profession. These organizations did not state explicitly that women were ineligible, but the available evidence reports the absence of female practitioners in the membership lists. The more inclusive nature of these county societies is reflected in the ratio of members to population. In contrast to the Massachusetts Medical Society with a ratio in 1781 of 1:5,657, Berkshire had 1:1,219, Middlesex 1:2,487, and Worcester 1:1,234.[88]

County societies were created to "eliminate the manifold inconveniences" that resulted from the "want of a regular and uniform method of educating pupils in physick, especially in the country." Yet, they, too, indirectly sought control over practice; for example, the Berkshire County Medical Association stipulated that if "Any person residing within the limits of this county [Berkshire], and pretending to practice physic and shall refuse . . . to become a member by attending the meetings and subscribing to the rules, . . . shall be treated with entire neglect by all that are members."[89] This open membership policy stands in contrast to the original intention of the state society to require all members to have a college education and an apprenticeship, "as it is in the mind of most of the Gentlemen of this town [Boston] never to vote for one that has not had one."[90] But the first president of the state society, Dr. Edward A. Holyoke, who possessed a bachelor's degree and apprenticeship training, did not believe that a college education should be a prerequisite for membership, nor did he "think it advisable to enjoin an Attendance on the medical lectures at Harvard," which were first offered in 1782, because it would be a "great inconvenience to many" living outside Boston and Cambridge.[91]

In some ways the regulatory ambitions of the Harvard Medical School, created in 1783, and the Massachusetts Medical Society, founded two years before, clashed.[92] Harvard produced M.D.s, but the society claimed the right to examine and certify them along with other, degreeless, practitioners. A similar situation obtained in London, where the Royal College of Physicians certified the graduates of medical schools in Scotland and England.

At the close of the eighteenth century, despite the appearance of new institutions, the regulation of medical practice differed little from what it had been in the seventeenth century. Although the "Great design" of the state medical society had been "to check the Growth of Imposters and lay a foundation for Improvement in Medical Knowledge," in practice, complained one member, the "institution of the Massachusetts Medical Society has not in the least degree prevented the Increase of Empirics."[93]

Boston doctors failed to centralize medical authority in Massachusetts, just as London practitioners failed to control medical practice in the provinces. But unlike the English guilds, which at least partially succeeded in regulating medical practice in London, the medical societies of Massachusetts had little to show for their efforts. In many ways the organization of medicine in Massachusetts, and in all of New England, resembled arrangements neither in London nor in the English provinces. In Massachusetts,

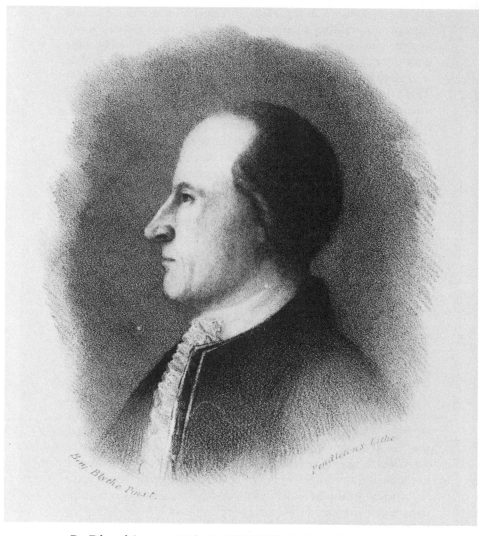

Dr. Edward Augustus Holyoke (1728-1829) of Salem, Massachusetts, graduated from Harvard College in 1749 and learned medicine as an apprentice. He served as mentor to dozens of medical pupils and, in 1781, became the first president of the Massachusetts Medical Society. Courtesy of the Francis A. Countway Library of Medicine.

where there were few degree-holding practitioners, the level of training was low and titles were employed indiscriminately; in London, or even in the provinces, "physicians" possessed M.D.s, regardless of their function. During the eighteenth century, however, just as the structure of medical practice in provincial England began more closely to resemble that in London, so too did the structure of practice in rural Massachusetts begin to bear similarities to that in Boston. The trend already evident in England toward formal academic training and certification for practice was also slowly gathering momentum in New England.

Medical Practice and Therapeutics

Although England had supported hospitals since the Middle Ages, few survived the Reformation. The beginnings of the voluntary hospital movement in the second quarter of the eighteenth century soon had parallels in the British colonies, beginning with the Philadelphia Hospital, which opened in 1751. Hospitals did not appear in New England, however, until the nineteenth century.[91] Several factors contributed to this delay. Only large towns and cities could afford to maintain a hospital, and during the colonial period New England remained predominantly rural. Besides, most immigrants came from provincial England and thus, unlike London residents, were unaccustomed to the presence of hospitals. Families and municipalities assumed responsibility for medical charity.[95] Finally, the apprenticeship system of training doctors encouraged practice in the homes of their patients.

The only "hospitals" in New England before 1800 were the alms-houses, pesthouses, and poorhouses found in the larger communities, such as Boston; the temporary facilities used for quarantine and inoculation during smallpox epidemics; and the military hospitals established during the several colonial wars.[96] Many of these institutions contracted with doctors on a year-to-year basis; at least 118 Massachusetts practitioners supplemented their income in this way. Sometimes the awarding of commissions to care for the indigent involved political considerations. In 1773, for example, Dr. Joseph Warren, a Harvard graduate with apprenticeship training, was replaced as physician to the Boston almshouse by a man of more "conservative politics," Dr. Samuel Danforth, who possessed similar medical credentials.[97]

Between 1764 and 1780, 73 percent of the ninety-two inoculators in Massachusetts worked in specially prepared isolation facilities rather than in the homes of their patients. During the War for Independence, Dr. Nathaniel Ames, Jr., a college graduate with apprenticeship training, earned a handsome fee for inoculating patients at the smallpox hospital in Marblehead, north of Boston.[98] Such public services were usually provided by the medical elite, who at least had served apprenticeships.[99]

Responsibility for medical care in New England, as in the mother country, often devolved upon the sick themselves or their families, who picked up the rudiments of medicine from a variety of sources, including self-help manuals, newspapers, almanacks, and even medical texts.[100] When families could not treat their own medical problems, they called in a neighbor or sought the advice of local persons reputed to have medical expertise: grocers, booksellers, midwives, nurses, bone setters, and ministers, as well as apothecaries, surgeons, and physicians.[101] Unfortunately, we know little about the activities of most of these practitioners.

Contemporary records suggest that male doctors did not challenge the monopoly of female midwives until after 1750. The most familiar names in the annals of colonial midwifery are those associated with the settlement of Boston in the 1630s: Anne Hutchinson and Jane Hawkins, who were exiled from the town for theological reasons, and Margaret Jones, who was executed for witchcraft in 1648.[102] The extent of some practices is indicated by the fact that Elizabeth Phillips, a London-certified midwife, delivered over 3,000 babies between 1719 and 1761.[103] Although most midwives worked as private practitioners in the homes of their clients, some were paid by local communities to serve prospective mothers who were unwed or who lived in the poorhouse.

During the early decades of the eighteenth century, Boston supported at least a dozen apothecary shops. Under the sign of the Unicorn & Mortar, Dr. Silvester Gardiner conducted what was perhaps the largest wholesale drug business in New England until the 1770s: importing herbs and chemicals, preparing medicines, and selling medical and surgical books and apparatus.[104] Some Boston doctors, like their London counterparts, may have relied upon apothecaries to prepare their prescriptions; but in most of the settlements around Massachusetts, as in provincial England, medical practitioners either prepared their own prescriptions or had their apprentices do it. A survey of 167 inventories of eighteenth-century doctors' estates reveals that over two-thirds contained a substantial quantity of herbs, chemicals, and instruments necessary for compounding prescriptions.[105] These estates also included London pharmacopoeias (standard lists of ingredients of commonly prescribed preparations).

The estate inventories also document that virtually every doctor owned a set of basic surgical instruments: lancets for bloodletting or opening abscesses and scalpels for removing superficial abnormalities. Most colonial practitioners, however, seem to have left excisions of large fleshy tumours, amputations of extremities, and lithotomies to medical men having the requisite anatomical and surgical training. Dr. Gardiner's success at performing lithotomies indicates that he was just as capable, if not as fast, as his mentor, William Cheselden in London.[106] Gardiner, Bulfinch, Sr., Zabdiel Boylston, and James Lloyd, among others in the Boston area, brought home from England and Europe the most advanced surgical techniques, and they, in turn, taught these to their many students who practiced in the colony.

Regarding his practice in Boston during the first half of the eighteenth century, the European-trained William Douglass confided that he could

> live handsomely here by the incomes of my practice, and save some small matter . . . here we have a great trade and many strangers with whom my business chiefly consists. I have a practice here among four sorts of People. . . .

His four types of patients were: (1) families that paid him an annual fee for his services, (2) occasional patients in need of immediate care, (3) poorhouse or "free" patients, and (4) native New Englanders from whom he had difficulty collecting fees.[107] The mobility of New Englanders produced many "strangers" not only in Boston but throughout the state. Douglass' account of his practice in Boston, though in some respects unique to large seacoast towns, was in many ways descriptive of medical practice throughout the region, and even in provincial England, although his reference to poorhouse patients differentiates his practice from the majority of his contemporaries. Douglass, who practiced primar-

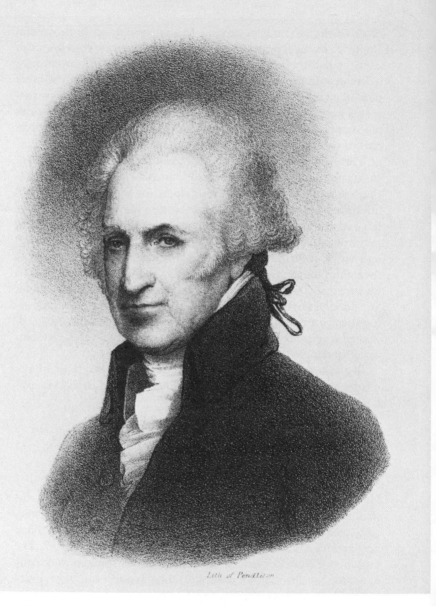

Dr. James Lloyd (1728-1810) of Boston completed an apprenticeship with a local practitioner before sailing for London, where he studied with some of the prominent English physicians of the time. By 1760 he was widely acknowledged as one of New England's most skilled and successful surgeons and a pioneer man-midwife. Courtesy of the Francis A. Countway Library of Medicine.

ily as a physician, did not prepare his own prescriptions, but he did assist in some surgical cases, thus demonstrating that even the best-trained doctors of New England combined the functions of Old World guilds.

Generalizations about therapeutics in New England before 1800 have often been based on William Douglass' description. Medical practice, he alleged, "was very uniform, bleeding, vomiting, blistering, purging, anodyne, etc., if the illness continued there was repetendi, and finally murderandi." Also, he claimed, his fellow New Englanders followed the English physician Sydenham "too much in giving paregoricks, after catharticks, which is playing fast and loose." According to Douglass, the most commonly used drugs, taken in "unbelievable quantities," were calomel (mercurous chloride), opium preparations (laudanum, paregoric), ipecac, Jesuit's bark (cinchona bark), and snake root.[108] The evidence in recent studies, however, fails to support his contention that most New England practitioners over-prescribed these drugs and that they dealt in "quackish medicines."

Analyses of over 7,000 patient visits made by five apprentice-trained New England doctors — three of whom practiced in New Hampshire and two in the Boston area — provide a radically different picture of colonial medical practice.[109] The ledger books of these doctors, covering the years 1770 to 1795, show that bleeding was prescribed for only about 7 percent of their patients. In 10 percent of their non-surgical cases, these doctors gave no drugs at all, only advice about diet and regimen. The most commonly prescribed medications, in order of frequency, were liquid laudanum, paregoric elixir, and ipecac (all 1 percent or less), cinchona bark (2.48 percent to 11 percent), calomel (less than 3 percent), and snakeroot and anodyne balsam (less than 4 percent). Although the native plants of New England were, in the opinion of one recent scholar, "insufficient to furnish most of the medical profession's therapeutic needs," all but one of the doctors used the "emetic weed" (*Lobelia inflata*), one of the "few native plants that found major use in early American medicine."[110] Of the 100 most commonly used ingredients, sixty-eight were botanical, twenty-six chemical or mineral, and six were derived from animal products. Nearly half of these substances were imported; many of the remainder came from native plants, but they constituted "only a small proportion of all the drugs administered."[111] All five doctors, regardless of their location, tended to follow uniform practices. Thus it seems that the heroic therapies described by Douglass were neither widely nor commonly administered.

When Dr. John Perkins visited London in 1734, he discovered great similarities between medical practice in the English city and that of Boston, and when, in 1777, he committed his recollection of that visit to paper, he evidently saw little reason to modify his original impressions. The actual practice of medicine, whether in treating gout, worms, dysentery, or broken bones, seems to have differed little between the colonies and the English provinces, or even London. New England medical practitioners admired and followed Sydenham's Hippocratic teachings to advise the patient of proper diet and fresh air, and to recognize the *vis medicatrix naturae* (the healing powers of nature). Experience-oriented as they were, these doctors did not produce new medical theories to replace those of the Old World, although some evidence suggests that they may have been more flexible and less harsh in their therapeutics than European authorities recommended. The successful New England experiments with controlled smallpox inoculation, which antedated similar developments in England by years, serves as the most obvious example of this tendency.

CONCLUSION

The differences between medical organizations, practice, and therapeutics in Old and New England during most of the seventeenth and eighteenth centuries cannot be attributed solely to climatic variations between the two regions. In 1623, Governor Edward Winslow, Jr., of Plymouth, observed:

> I can scarce distinguish New England from Old England in respect of heat and cold. . . . Some object because our plantation lieth in the latitude of 42 degrees it must needs be much hotter. I confess I cannot give the reason of the contrary; only experience teacheth us that if it do exceed England, it is so little as must require better judgements to discern it.[112]

Emphasizing the similarities that he observed at the time, William Wood wrote in 1639 that "onions and whatever grows well in England" also flourished in New England soil.[113]

The absence of guild restrictions, together with the presence of rapid demographic change, did not produce a unique form of medical thought and action among New Englanders. The institutional and intellectual environment of the New World was not sufficiently different from that of the Old World to produce more than variations in degree. The blurring of medical functions was widespread in provincial England as well as in America; both regions were moving in the same direction but at different rates of speed. English controversies over functions and titles, such as "physician," were similar in many respects to the debates in Massachusetts concerning the training appropriate for the title of "doctor." In their attempts to modify or eliminate medical traditions, reformers in both areas failed to reach a consensus regarding the necessity of academic and practical training. As the historian Michael Kammen has observed, the professions in England were not as highly developed as we have assumed, "nor were they so primitive in provincial America as some had suspected."[114]

NOTES

I wish to thank Professor Harold J. Cook, Department of the History of Medicine, University of Wisconsin-Madison, for reading a draft of this essay and making valuable critical remarks. His book, *The Decline of the Old Medical Regime in Stuart London* (Ithaca, N.Y.: Cornell Univ. Press, 1986), is a major contribution to our understanding of seventeenth-century medicine in England. I also wish to express appreciation to Darlene Mickey and Dottie Leathers for preparing the typescript.

1. In particular, Daniel J. Boorstin, *The Americans: The Colonial Experience* (New York: Vintage, 1958). A brief, penetrating analysis of the historiography of such comparative efforts is Hugh Kearney, "The Problem of Perspective in the History of Colonial America," in K.R. Andrews, N.P. Canny, and P.E.H. Hair, eds., *The Westward Enterprise: English Activities in Ireland, the Atlantic, and America, 1480–1650* (Detroit: Wayne State Univ. Press, 1979), 290–302. The quotation is from John Perkins, "Memoirs of the Life Writings and Opinions of John Perkins Physician lately of Boston. begun March. 1777. and continued to 1778," manuscript memoirs, American Antiquarian Society, Worcester, Mass. (with permission of the Society), 2.

2. D.B. Quinn, *England and the Discovery of America, 1481–1620* (New York: Knopf, 1974).

3. E.A. Wrigley and R.S. Schofield, *The Population History of England, 1541–1871* (Cambridge, Mass.: Harvard Univ. Press, 1981).

4. H.C. Darby, ed., *A New Historical Geography of England* (Cambridge: Univ. of Cambridge Press, 1973), 293–98, 381, 459.

5. Thomas H. Breen and Stephen Foster, "The Way to the New World: The Character of Early Massachusetts Immigration," *William and Mary Quarterly*, 3rd ser. (1973), 30:189–222.

6. Ernest Caulfield, "Some Common Diseases of Colonial Children," Colonial Society of Massachusetts, *Transactions* (1942–46), 25:4–65, 36.

7. Charles Creighton, *A History of Epidemics in Great Britain*, 2 vols., 2nd ed. (New York: Barnes and Noble, 1965), I:646–92; William H. McNeill, *Plagues and Peoples* (Garden City, N.Y.: Anchor Books, 1976), 152; Frederick W. Cartwright, *Disease and History* (New York: Crowell, 1972), 121–22, 132–33.

8. Quoted in Owen H. and Sara D. Wangensteen, *The Rise of Surgery from Empiric Craft to Scientific Discipline* (Minneapolis: Univ. of Minnesota Press, 1978), 65.

9. Cartwright, *Disease and History*, 132; and John Duffy, *Epidemics in Colonial America* (Baton Rouge: Louisiana State Univ. Press, 1953), 165.

10. J. Worth Estes, *Hall Jackson and the Purple Foxglove: Medical Practice and Research in Revolutionary America, 1760–1820* (Hanover: Univ. Press of New England, 1979), 131.

11. On medical institutions, practices, and personnel, see, e.g., Sir George Clark, *A History of the Royal College of Physicians of London* (Oxford: Clarendon Press, 1964); Zachary Cope, *The Royal College of Surgeons of England* (Springfield, Ill.: Charles C. Thomas, 1959); Josephine A. Dolan, *History of Nursing*, 12th ed. (Philadelphia: W.B. Saunders, 1969); F.N.L. Poynter, ed., *The Evolution of Medical Practice in Britain* (London: Pitman Medical Publishing Co., 1961); John L. Thornton, ed., *James R. Aveling's English Midwives*, 1872 (London: Hugh K. Elliot Ltd., 1967); and E. Ashworth Underwood, ed., *A History of the Worshipful Society of Apothecaries of London*, 2 vols. (London: Oxford Univ. Press, 1963), I:1617–1815.

12. Quoted in John A. Raach, "Five Early Seventeenth Century English Country Physicians," *Journal of the History of Medicine and Allied Sciences* (1965), 20:213.

13. Margaret Pelling, "Occupational Diversity: Barbersurgeons and the Trades of Norwich, 1550–1640, *Bulletin of the History of Medicine* (1982), 56:484–511, esp. 489; and Pelling and Charles Webster, "Medical Practitioners," in Charles Webster, ed., *Health, Medicine and Mortality in the Sixteenth Century* (Cambridge: Cambridge Univ. Press, 1979), 165–235, esp. 165–68.

14. Surgical developments for the period are discussed in William N. Boog Watson, "Four Monopolies and the Surgeons of London and Edinburgh," *Journal of the History of Medicine and Allied Sciences*

(1970), 25:311–22; Lloyd G. Stevenson, "A Note on the Relation of Military Service to Licensing in the History of British Surgery," *Bulletin of the History of Medicine* (1953), 27:420–27; Richard Hardaway Meade, *An Introduction to the History of General Surgery* (Philadelphia: W.B. Saunders, 1968); and Wangensteen and Wangensteen, *The Rise of Surgery*.

15. Pelling and Webster, "Medical Practitioners," 182–84.

16. The changing prospects for apothecaries and for other types of practitioners in urban and rural areas are discussed in Sir Humphrey Rolleston, "History of Medicine in the City of London," *Annals of Medical History* (1941), 3:1–17; Pelling, "Occupational Diversity"; Pelling and Webster, "Medical Practitioners"; John R. Guy, "The Episcopal Licensing of Physicians, Surgeons and Midwives," *Bulletin of the History of Medicine* (1982), 56:528–42; Thomas R. Forbes, "Apprentices in Trouble: The Training of Surgeons and Apothecaries," *Yale Journal of Biology and Medicine* (1979), 52:227–37; J.J. Keevil, "The Seventeenth Century English Medical Background," *Bulletin of the History of Medicine* (1957), 31:408–24; and R.S. Roberts, "The Personnel and Practice of Medicine in Tudor and Stuart England," *Medical History* (1962), 6:363–82; and (1964), 8:217–34.

17. Lester S. King, *The Medical World of the Eighteenth Century* (Chicago: Univ. of Chicago Press, 1958), 18–29, and Rolleston, "Medicine in London," 4–6.

18. See, e.g., A.J. Rook, "Cambridge Medical Students at Leyden," *Medical History* (1973), 27:256–65; and R.W. Innes-Smith, *English-Speaking Students of Medicine at the University of Leyden* (Edinburgh: Oliver and Boyd, 1932).

19. Gweneth Whitteridge and Veronica Stokes, *A Brief History of the Hospital of Saint Bartholomew* (London: Brown, Knight & Truscott Ltd., 1961); Pelling and Webster, "Medical Practitioners," 180–81; and Susan C. Lawrence, "'Desirous of Improvements in Medicine': Pupils and Practitioners in the Medical Societies at Guy's and St. Bartholomew's Hospitals, 1795–1815," *Bulletin of the History of Medicine* (1985), 59:89–104.

20. Pelling, "Occupational Diversity," 189–90; and Pelling and Webster, "Medical Practitioners," 165, 233–35.

21. Joseph F. Kett, "Provincial Medical Practice in England, 1730–1815," *Journal of the History of Medicine and Allied Sciences* (1964), 19:17–29.

22. Ibid., 27.

23. Guy, "Episcopal Licensing," 529–37.

24. Kett, "Provincial Practice," 26–29; and Ivan Waddington, "The Struggle to Reform the Royal College of Physicians, 1767–1771: A Sociological Analysis," *Medical History* (1973), 17:107–26.

25. Pelling and Webster, "Medical Practitioners," 225–27.

26. Ibid., 215.

27. Pelling, "Occupational Diversity," 508; and Leslie G. Matthews, "Licensed Mountebanks in Britain," *Journal of the History of Medicine and Allied Sciences* (1964), 19:30–45.

28. Pelling, "Occupational Diversity," 498, 507–508.

29. Pelling and Webster, "Medical Practitioners," 188.

30. The data in this section are derived from John A. Raach, *A Directory of English Country Physicians, 1603–1643* (London: Dawson's of Pall Mall, 1962).

31. Pelling and Webster, "Medical Practitioners," 232.

32. Ibid., 235. Later, in "Occupational Diversity," page 508, Pelling would increase the ratio to 1:200, suggesting also that the "true ratio may well be higher."

33. The basic sources here are A. Batty Shaw, "The Oldest Medical Societies in Great Britain," *Medical History* (1968), 12:232–44, and Lawrence, "Desirous of Improvements."

34. Lawrence, "Desirous of Improvements," 91 n. 12.

35. Ibid., 89.

36. Ibid., 101.

37. Walter Radcliffe, "The Colchester Medical Society, 1774," *Medical History* (1976), 20:394–401.

38. Owsei Temkin, *Galenism: Rise and Decline of a Medical Philosophy* (Ithaca, N.Y.: Cornell Univ. Press, 1973), and Wesley D. Smith, *The Hippocratic Tradition* (Ithaca, N.Y.: Cornell Univ. Press, 1979).

39. Stanley Joel Reiser, *Medicine and the Reign of Technology* (Cambridge: Cambridge Univ. Press, 1978), 1–22.

40. Walter Pagel, *Paracelsus: An Introduction to Philosophical Medicine in the Era of the Renaissance* (New York: S. Karger, 1958); and Webster, "Alchemical and Paracelsian Medicine," in *Health, Medicine, and Mortality,* 301–34.

41. Reiser, *Reign of Technology,* 8–10; and Lester S. King, *The Growth of Medical Thought* (Chicago: Univ. of Chicago Press, 1963; Midway Reprint, 1973), 19.

42. Raach, "Country Physicians," 218.

43. Because of the great variety of medical assistance available in London and in provincial cities and towns, no definitive generalization can be made at this time (Pelling and Webster, "Medical Practitioners," 233–34). Major surgical intervention may have been an exception. Patients requiring extensive surgical treatment may have been encouraged to avoid the traveling lithotomist and to seek instead the practitioners in larger towns, like Norwich. The emergence of one provincial town as a regional center

for risky operations is detailed in A. Batty Shaw, "The Norwich School of Lithotomy," *Medical History* (1970), *14*:228–59.

44. Nicholas Canny, "The Permissive Frontier: The Problem of Social Control in English Settlements in Ireland and Virginia, 1550–1650," 17–44, and Karl S. Bottigheimer, "Kingdom and Colony: Ireland in the Westward Enterprise, 1536–1660," 45–64, in Andrews, Canny, and Hair, eds., *Westward Enterprise*.

45. Evarts B. Greene and Virginia D. Harrington, *American Population Before the Federal Census of 1790* (New York: Columbia Univ. Press, 1932); and U.S. Bureau of the Census, *Historical Statistics of the United States: Colonial Times to 1957* (Washington, D.C.: U.S. Government Printing Office, 1961).

46. Ralph J. Crandall, "New England's Second Great Migration: The First Three Generations of Settlement, 1630–1700," *The New England Historical and Genealogical Register* (1975), *129*:347–60; and Breen and Foster, "Early Massachusetts Immigration," 189–222.

47. Darrett B. Rutman, *Winthrop's Boston: A Portrait of a Puritan Town* (Chapel Hill: Univ. of North Carolina Press, 1965); Edmund S. Morgan, *The Puritan Dilemma: The Story of John Winthrop* (Boston: Little, Brown, 1958); and Crandall, "Second Great Migration," 359.

48. Morgan, *Puritan Dilemma*, 120–33; and Sumner Chilton Powell, *A Puritan Village* (Middletown: Wesleyan Univ. Press, 1963).

49. Eric H. Christianson, "The Emergence of Medical Communities in Massachusetts, 1700–1794: The Demographic Factors," *Bulletin of the History of Medicine* (1980), *54*:64–77, esp. 66.

50. John Demos, *A Little Commonwealth: Family Life in Plymouth Colony* (New York: Oxford Univ. Press, 1970); and Philip J. Greven, *Four Generations: Population, Land, and Family in Colonial Andover, Massachusetts* (New York: Norton, 1970).

51. This section is based on Duffy, *Colonial Epidemics*; Caulfield, "Common Diseases"; John B. Blake, *Public Health in the Town of Boston, 1630–1822* (Cambridge, Mass.: Harvard Univ. Press, 1959); James H. Cassedy, "Meteorology and Medicine in Colonial America: Beginnings of the Experimental Approach," *Journal of the History of Medicine and Allied Sciences* (1969), *24*:193–204; James H. Cassedy, "Church Record-Keeping and Public Health in Early New England," in Philip Cash, Eric H. Christianson, and J. Worth Estes, eds., *Medicine in Colonial Massachusetts, 1620–1820*, Publications of the Colonial Society of Massachusetts, v. 57 (distributed by the Univ. of Virginia Press, 1980), 249–62; Rose S. Lockwood, "Birth, Illness and Death in Eighteenth-Century New England," *Journal of Social History* (1978), *12*:111–28; and Otho T. Beall, Jr., and Richard H. Shryock, *Cotton Mather: First Signifi-*

cant Figure in American Medicine (Baltimore: Johns Hopkins Press, 1954).

52. Medical practitioners and community leaders were often the same individuals, whose medical advice reflected local political alignments. Dennis Don Melchert, "Experimenting on the Neighbors: Inoculation of Smallpox in Boston in the Context of Eighteenth Century Medicine" (unpubl. Ph.D. diss., Univ. of Iowa, 1973).

53. For purposes of comparison, Whitfield J. Bell, Jr., "A Portrait of the Colonial Physician," *Bulletin of the History of Medicine* (1970), 44:497–517; Wyndham B. Blanton, *Medicine in Virginia in the Eighteenth Century* (Richmond: Garrett and Massie, 1931); David L. Cowan, *Medicine and Health in New Jersey: A History* (New Brunswick, N.J.: Rutgers Univ. Press, 1964); Maurice Bear Gordon, *Aesculapius Comes to the Colonies: The Story of the Early Days of Medicine in the Thirteen Original Colonies* (Ventor, N.J.: Ventor Publishers, 1949); Jonathan Harris, "The Rise of Medical Science in New York, 1720–1820" (unpubl. Ph.D. diss., New York Univ., 1971); Joseph F. Kett, *The Formation of the American Medical Profession: The Role of Institutions, 1780–1860* (New Haven, Conn.: Yale Univ. Press, 1968); William Frederick Norwood, *Medical Education in the United States Before the Civil War* (Philadelphia: Univ. of Pennsylvania Press, 1944); Francis R. Packard, *The History of Medicine in the United States*, 2 vols. (New York: Hafner, 1963); Byron Stookey, *A History of Colonial Medical Education in the Province of New York, With Its Subsequent Development, 1767–1830* (Springfield, Ill.: Charles C. Thomas, 1962); Joseph M. Toner, *Contributions to the Annals of Medical Progress and Medical Education in the United States Before and During the War of Independence* (Washington, D.C.: U.S. Government Printing Office, 1874); and Joseph Ivor Waring, *A History of Medicine in South Carolina, 1670–1825* (Charleston: South Carolina Medical Association, 1964).

54. Christianson, "The Medical Practitioners of Massachusetts 1630–1800: Patterns of Change and Continuity," in Cash, Christianson, and Estes, eds., *Medicine in Colonial Massachusetts,* 49–67, esp. 57; and C.H. Brock and Eric H. Christianson, "Appendix: A Biographical Register of Men and Women from and Immigrants to Massachusetts between 1620 and 1800 Who Received Some Medical Training in Europe," in Cash, Christianson, and Estes, eds., *Medicine in Colonial Massachusetts,* 117–43.

55. Christianson, "Medical Practitioners," 52–54, 65–66; Samuel A. Green, *History of Medicine in Massachusetts* (Boston: A. Williams and Company, 1881), 15; and Henry R. Viets, *A Brief History of Medicine in Massachusetts* (Boston: Houghton Mifflin, 1930), 11–12.

56. The information about these four men is from my unpublished

manuscript, "The Tachygraphy of Dr. Jasper Gunn (1606–1671)"; and Malcolm Sydney Beinfield, "The Early New England Doctor: An Adaptation to A Provincial Environment," *Yale Journal of Biology and Medicine* (1942–43), *15*:99–132, 271–88.

57. Kett, "Provincial England."

58. The act is quoted in Richard H. Shryock, *Medical Licensing in America, 1650–1965* (Baltimore: Johns Hopkins Press, 1967), p. vii.

59. Christianson, "Medical Practitioners," 52–54. On the underestimation of practitioners by earlier studies, see Christianson, "The Historiography of Early American Medicine," in Cash, Christianson, and Estes, eds., *Medicine in Colonial Massachusetts,* 20–25. The estimations in the present study are derived primarily from a systematic analysis of the vital records (births, deaths, and marriages), and histories of some 300 Massachusetts towns and eleven counties. Women practitioners and midwives were not generally reported in vital records; studies of court records may identify many of them, and nurses as well. Future research will undoubtedly identify more practitioners that will produce higher ratios.

60. Ibid., 54–55.

61. Toner, *Annals of Progress,* 105–106; and Shryock, *Medicine and Society,* 12.

62. Kett, *Institutions,* 170, and Christianson, "Medical Communities," 69–70.

63. The material on the Bulfinches is based on Edward Jacob Forster, "A Sketch of the Medical Profession of Suffolk County," in *The Professional and Industrial History of Suffolk County, Massachusetts in Three Volumes* (Boston: Boston History Company, 1881), III:259; Francis R. Packard, "Cheselden's American Pupils," *Annals of Medical History* (1937), *9*:533–48, esp. 536; Edgar M. Bick, "French Influences in Early American Medicine and Surgery," *Journal of Mt. Sinai Hospital* (1957), *24*:499–509; Rolleston, "Medicine in London," 11–16; Charles Coury, "L'Hôtel Dieu de Paris, un des plus anciens hopiteaux d' Europe," *Medical History Journal* (1967), *2*:269–316; Clifford K. Shipton, *Sibley's Harvard Graduates . . . ,* 17 vols. to date (Boston: Massachusetts Historical Society, 1933–), *XII*:16–23; Dr. William Cullen's manuscript list of "Students in the College of Chemistry, 1755–1765" (Univ. of Edinburgh Library); Lewis, "American Graduates"; and Christianson, "Individuals in the Healing Arts and the Emergence of a Medical Community in Massachusetts, 1700–1792: A Collective Biography" (unpubl. Ph.D. diss., Univ. of Southern California, 1976), 84–85.

64. Whitfield J. Bell, Jr., "Medicine in Boston and Philadelphia: Comparisons and Contrasts, 1750–1820," and "Appendix: New England Stu-

dents at the Pennsylvania Hospital from the Revolution to 1820," in Cash, Christianson, and Estes, eds., *Medicine in Colonial Massachusetts,* 159–83.

65. Brock and Christianson, "Biographical Register"; and Christianson, "Medical Practitioners," 56–57.

66. Lewis, "American Graduates," 159–65.

67. William Pepper, *The Medical Side of Benjamin Franklin* (Philadelphia: W.J. Campbell, 1911), 41–44. Like John Perkins, Waterhouse did not find much difference in the practice of general medicine in Europe, England, or by then, the U.S.

68. Christianson, "Medical Practitioners," 57.

69. BMS misc. papers, with the permission of the Francis A. Countway Library of Medicine, Boston. This agreement is also quoted in Henry R. Viets, "The Medical Education of James Lloyd in Colonial America," *Yale Journal of Biology and Medicine* (1958), 31:1–13, esp. 6–7. Other agreements are cited and discussed in Genevieve Miller, "Medical Apprenticeship in the American Colonies," *Ciba Symposia* (1947), 8:502–10. For a discussion of medical pupils who paid a flat fee rather than served as apprentices, see Christianson, "Medical Practitioners," 52 n. 8.

70. Perkins, "Life Writings and Opinions," 2, 3, 71. He studied with Dr. William Davis in 1718 and Dr. Francis Archibald in 1721, both of Boston.

71. Christianson, "Medical Communities," 69, and Christianson, "Individuals in the Healing Arts," 114–16.

72. This section is based on Christianson, "Individuals in the Healing Arts," 85–116; Christianson, "Medical Communities," 69; and Christianson, "Medical Practitioners," 57–58.

73. Edward J. Young, "Subjects for Master's Degrees in Harvard College from 1655 to 1791," *Proceedings, Massachusetts Historical Society* (1880), 18:119–51; and Christianson, "Individuals in the Healing Arts," 88–92.

74. This section is based on my unpublished manuscript, "'In Case he inclines to follow a Doctor's Calling': The Role of the Medical Family in the Training of Early American Doctors"; and Christianson, "Individuals in the Healing Arts," 73.

75. Radcliffe, "Colchester Medical Society"; Shaw, "Oldest Medical Societies"; and Christianson, "Individuals in the Healing Arts," 155–88.

76. Uncatalogued Silvester Gardiner Papers, courtesy of the Francis A. Countway Library of Medicine, Boston; and Eric H. Christianson, "The Colonial Surgeon's Rise to Prominence: Dr. Silvester Gardiner (1707–1786), and the Practice of Lithotomy in New England," *The New England Historical and Genealogical Register* (1982), 136:104–14.

77. The standard account is George H. Weaver, "Life and Writings of William Douglass, M.D. (1691–1752)," *Bulletin of the Society of Medical History of Chicago* (1921), 9:229–59.

78. *The Boston Weekly News-Letter,* Dec. 29, 1737–Jan. 5, 1738.

79. G.B. Warden, "The Medical Profession in Colonial Boston," in Cash, Christianson, and Estes, eds., *Medicine in Colonial Massachusetts,* 145–59, argues that without a legal monopoly, medical societies were hopeless as agencies of control.

80. "An Elegy on the Death of the Late Dr. Ames," in Nathaniel Ames, *An Astronomical Diary; or Almanack, for . . . 1765* (Boston: Draper, Edes & Gill, Green & Russell, and Fleet, 1764), n.p.

81. Quoted in Walter A. Burrage, *A History of the Massachusetts Medical Society with Brief Biographies of the Founders and Chief Officers, 1781–1922* (privately printed, 1923), 3–7.

82. Christianson, "Individuals in the Healing Arts," 168–73.

83. Shipton, *Sibley's Harvard Graduates,* XV:3–15; Sarah Breck Baker, "Extracts from the Ames Diary," *Dedham Historical Register* (1890–1903), 1:9, 2:24, 59, 60, 148, 150; John Morgan, *A Discourse upon the Institution of Medical Schools in America* (Philadelphia, 1765), 24. For a discussion of Morgan's ideas, see Toby Gelfand, "The Origins of a Modern Concept of Medical Specialization: John Morgan's *Discourse* of 1765," *Bulletin of the History of Medicine* (1976), 50:511–35.

84. See, e.g., Philip Cash, *Medical Men at the Siege of Boston, April, 1775–April, 1776* (Philadelphia: American Philosophical Society, 1973).

85. Quoted in W.B. McDaniel, II, "A Letter from Dr. Williams Smibert of Boston, to his Former Fellow-Student at Edinburgh, Dr. John Morgan, of Philadelphia, Written February 14, 1769," *Annals of Medical History* (1939), 1:194–96.

86. Burrage, *Massachusetts Medical Society,* 16, 68–84, 323–49.

87. Ibid., 181–82.

88. Christianson, "Medical Communities," 75.

89. Manuscript Records of the Berkshire District Medical Society, 1785–1864, Berkshire Athenaeum, Pittsfield, p. 4.

90. Nathaniel Walker Appleton to Edward A. Holyoke, 9 June 1782, Holyoke Family Papers, MSS49, Essex Institute, Box 16, Folder 2.

91. Edward A. Holyoke to Nathaniel Walker Appleton, 18 April 1789, ibid., Folder 3.

92. Burrage, *Massachusetts Medical Society,* chs. 2, 3, 10; Kett, *Institutions,* 15; and Thomas F. Harrington, *The Harvard Medical School: A History, Narrative and Documentary,* 3 vols. (New York: Lewis, 1905), I.

93. Ebenezer Hunt to Dr. Samuel Danforth, 13 October 1789 (BMS b. 75.1 F76); and Israel Atherton to Nathaniel Appleton Walker, 20 Oc-

tober 1789 (BMS b. 75.1 F723), courtesy of the Francis A. Countway Library of Medicine, Boston.

94. Bell, "Medicine in Boston and Philadelphia," 163–64.

95. Christianson, "Medical Practitioners," 52; and Douglas Lamar Jones, "Charity, Medical Charity, and Dependency in Eighteenth-Century Essex County, Massachusetts," in Cash, Christianson, and Estes, *Medicine in Massachusetts*, 199–213. Other informative works discussing medical charity are Shryock, *Medicine and Society*, 104–107; and Shaw, "The Norwich School of Lithotomy," 223–26.

96. Shipton, *Sibley's Harvard Graduates*, XIII:380–89.

97. Ibid., XII: 512–27; and John H. Cary, *Joseph Warren: Physician, Politician, Patriot* (Urbana: Univ. of Illinois Press, 1961), 31.

98. Shipton, *Sibley's Harvard Graduates*, XV:3–15.

99. Christianson, "Medical Communities," 70; and Christianson, "Individuals in the Healing Arts," 118, 131, 151.

100. George E. Gifford, Jr., "Botanic Remedies in Colonial Massachusetts, 1620–1820," in Cash, Christianson, and Estes, eds., *Medicine in Colonial Massachusetts*, 263–88; Wayland D. Hand, *Magical Medicine: The Folkloric Component of Medicine in the Folk Belief, Customs, and Rituals of the Peoples of Europe and America* (Berkeley: Univ. of California Press, 1980); Guenter B. Risse, Ronald L. Numbers, and Judith Walzer Leavitt, eds., *Medicine Without Doctors: Home Health Care in American History* (New York: Science History Publications, 1977); Otho T. Beall, Jr., "Aristotle's MASTERPIECE in America: A Landmark in the Folklore of Medicine," *William and Mary Quarterly*, 3rd ser. (1963), 20:207–22; and Christianson, "The Description and Treatment of the Fly-Blown Ear: An Aspect of Science and Medicine in Colonial America," *The Melsheimer Entomological Series* (1979), 26:1–12.

101. Few would doubt that, from the earliest settlements, local ministers also engaged in medical activities in the absence of trained medical personnel.

102. Green, *Massachusetts*, 2–32; Viets, *Brief History*, 14–40; and Jones, "Charity," 207–208.

103. Green, *Massachusetts*, 55.

104. Christianson, "Lithotomy in New England," 107.

105. Christianson, "Individuals in the Healing Arts," 143–45, 150.

106. Christianson, "Lithotomy in New England," 106, 108, 110.

107. Douglass to Dr. Cadwallader Colden, 20 February 1720/1, in "Letters from Dr. William Douglass to Cadwallader Colden of New York," *Collections*, Massachusetts Historical Society (1854), 2:164–89, esp. 165–66.

108. The quotations from Douglass are found in Duffy, *Epidemics*, 8. Douglass' description is endorsed by Shryock, *Medicine and Society*,

17, 19; Bell, "A Portrait of the Colonial Physician," *Bulletin of the History of Medicine* (1970), 44:497–517; and Malcolm Sydney Beinfield, "The Early New England Doctor."

109. Eotoo, *Hall Jackoon;* and J. Worth Eotoo, "Thorapoutio Praotioo in Colonial New England," in Cash, Christianson, and Estes, *Medicine in Colonial Massachusetts,* 289–383. Dr. Estes has extended this uniformity of practice into the nineteenth century in his article, "Naval Medicine in the Age of Sail: The Voyage of the *New York,* 1802–1803," *Bulletin of the History of Medicine* (1982), 56:238–53.

110. Estes, "Therapeutic Practice," 338, 344.

111. Ibid., 344–45.

112. Quoted in John A. Goodwin, *The Pilgrim Republic* (Boston: Houghton Mifflin, 1920), 581.

113. William Wood, *New England's Prospect . . . ,* 3rd ed. (London, 1639; Boston: Fleet, Green & Russell, 1764), 15. These observations have been confirmed by J.I. Falconer, *History of Agriculture in the Northern United States, 1620–1860* (1925; rpt. Clifton, N.J.: Augustus M. Kelley Publishers, 1973), 16, 99.

114. Michael Kammen, *People of Paradox: An Inquiry Concerning the Origins of American Civilization* (New York: Vintage, 1973), 28–29.

Conclusion

RONALD L. NUMBERS

The three case studies in this volume not only trace the transit of medicine from the Old World to the New, but provide an empirical basis for resolving the debate over the influence of the American environment on medical institutions and practices. As Guenter B. Risse has shown, medicine in New Spain closely mirrored medicine in Old Spain, which in the sixteenth century was ruled by a strong monarchy intent on exploiting the mineral and human resources of its new lands. During the century following Columbus' arrival in the New World in 1492, bureaucratic Spanish officials, aided by representatives of the Catholic church, successfully transplanted virtually all of the medical institutions found in Spain: the *protomedicato* to regulate the practice of medicine, hospitals to care for the sick, and medical professorships to train new physicians.[1]

For the most part, these transplanted institutions continued to function just as they had in Spain, adapting themselves only in minor ways to their new setting. Despite the shortage of qualified physicians and surgeons, the *protomedicato* continued to insist — with mixed results — on proper credentials and ethnic purity and to ban the practice of Aztec medicine. And instead of gradually succumbing to the liberalizing influence of the New World, the *protomedicato* actually stiffened its control of medicine in the mid-seventeenth century. Although many of the hospitals in New Spain took on a role that appears to be a novel accommodation to the needs of the New World—the conversion and acculturation of the Indians—this development merely perpetuated the long-standing Spanish practice of using hospitals to convert and acculturate such minority groups as the Moors. Regardless of the practical needs of a rough-and-tumble frontier community, medical students in Mexico City read the same books and mastered the same body of classical knowledge that students in Salamanca did.

The practice of medicine in New Spain also remained surprisingly static. Although the discovery of indigenous medical plants led to some additions to the pharmacopoeia, medical theory and practice scarcely changed. Instead of relying on expensive and sometimes scarce European drugs to induce vomiting, sweating, and evacuation of the bowels, the medical men of New Spain simply substituted comparable herbal remedies borrowed from the Aztecs; they neither revised their humoral pathology nor abandoned their depletive therapies.[2]

Unlike the Spanish, who stumbled onto a thriving civilization and temperate climate in Central America, the French colonists a century later took possession of a sparsely populated and relatively inhospitable land in present-day eastern Canada. Nevertheless, as Toby Gelfand has shown, the French, too, attempted to replant their basic medical structures in the New World during the years between the founding of Quebec in 1608 and the British conquest of 1760. The organization of medical care in Quebec and Montreal may have remained a pale imitation of that in Paris, but it bore a striking resemblance to what prevailed in the French provinces. In both colonial and provincial France apprentice-trained surgeons rather than university-educated physicians provided the bulk of the medical care, although, apparently in response to local conditions, the practitioners of New France seem to have possessed fewer skills, less power (for example, over midwives), and greater social mobility than their counterparts in the mother country.[3] It is true that medical guilds and societies failed to take root on this side of the Atlantic, but this seems to have resulted less from the democratizing effects of the environment than from the dominant position of the military and the church in New France. Besides, as Gelfand has reminded us, even in France the pyramidical structure of medicine had already become unstable. The absence of guilds, however, did not mean that medicine in New France went unregulated. Like the *protomédico* in Mexico City, the king's physician in Quebec determined who was, and was not, eligible to practice medicine.

Except for ministering to a somewhat broader spectrum of society and perhaps healing more of their patients, the hospitals of New France operated in the manner of provincial hospitals in France, just as colonial surgeons treated their patients with the same therapies administered to the sick in the mother country. Although the practitioners of New France, like their peers in New Spain, sometimes replaced traditional remedies with indigenous ones, they, too, held firmly to the therapeutic categories and procedures of the Old World. Thus, although the environment of New France slightly altered the ways in which medicine was organized and practiced, it failed to change the basic patterns of medical care.

The medical histories of New Spain and New France demonstrate that European institutions—regulatory agencies, hospitals, and medical schools—could survive in the New World and suggest that their absence in colonial New England resulted more from cultural than environmental factors. We also learn from the histories of colonies to the north and south of the English settlements that conditions of life in the New World did not automatically break down professional distinctions or lead to a rejection of traditional beliefs and practices. Thus it should come as no surprise that Eric Christianson, too, has stressed the commonality of medical practice in New England and in the nonurban areas of Great Britain, where general medical practice was commonplace. Moreover, he has shown how relationships between doctors in rural Massachusetts and in Boston mimicked those between practitioners in the British provinces and the London elite. And he has detected parallel movements in Old and New England during the eighteenth century to establish formal academic requirements for practicing medicine. Instead of diverging more and more from English models, medical institutions and practice in New England tended to become increasingly English as the years passed.

New Englanders did, however, modify some of the medical customs of the Old World. More than their relatives back home, they tended to call all medical men "doctors," regardless of their training.[4] And because of the pressing need for medical personnel and the lack of a centralized medical authority, neither of which was unique to New England, they reduced the average length of a medical apprenticeship—in practice, if not in theory—from a nominal seven years for apothecaries in England to little more than one year in Massachusetts, a finding that necessitates revising all previous estimates about the length of the colonial apprenticeship.[5] Christianson also tells us that colonial doctors practiced a milder form of medicine than we have previously been led to believe. Whatever the reasons for this, there is little ground for thinking that it resulted from any peculiarly American tendency toward innovation in the absence of Old World traditions and restrictions. In this regard it is instructive to recall that Cotton Mather's much-celebrated experiments with inoculation for smallpox in the early 1720s owed less to "a strong, if crude, empirical strain, a carelessness of theory, and an insistence on results," as Daniel J. Boorstin would have us believe, than to Mather's having read the *Philosophical Transactions* of the Royal Society of London, the leading scientific publication in the English-speaking world, which had favorably discussed inoculation several years earlier.[6]

Taken together, the studies of medicine in New Spain, New France, and New England allow us to draw several conclusions about medicine in the New World. Although most medical men in the colonies engaged in some form of general practice, this custom cannot be attributed to either the physical or social environments of North and Central America; general practice also typified medical care in the provincial regions of the Old World, which, as Richard H. Shryock noted years ago, supplied the colonies with most of their immigrants. The distinctive use of the *protomedicato* in New Spain, the prevalence of surgeons in New France, and the dominance of surgeon-apothecaries in New England are all traceable to traditions in the respective mother countries; they did not result from any occult environmental influences prevailing on the western shores of the Atlantic Ocean.

We also know that medical practice changed remarkably little in transit from the established societies of the Old World to the new settlements in the Americas. Medical practitioners in New Spain, New France and New England may have borrowed at times from indigenous healers and incorporated some native remedies into their pharmacopoeias, but their theoretical framework and their actual practices remained virtually unchanged. Even when they prescribed novel medicines, they did so for the same reasons that had governed Western medical practice for centuries. It would take more than a new environment to change old habits.

NOTES

1. Lycurgo de Castro Santos Filho has alluded to similar continuities in the history of medicine in New Portugal (present-day Brazil); see his "Medicine in Colonial Brazil: An Overview," in *Aspects of the History of Medicine in Latin America*, ed. John Z. Bowers and Elizabeth F. Purcell (New York: Josiah Macy, Jr. Foundation, 1979), 97–111.

2. This conclusion contradicts Gordon Schendel's assertion that Aztec and Spanish practices fused into a "unique" medical tradition; see Schendel, *Medicine in Mexico: From Aztec Herbs to Betatrons* (Austin: Univ. of Texas Press, 1968), 87.

3. In "If Turner Had Looked at Canada, Australia, and New Zealand When He Wrote about the West," in *The Frontier in Perspective*, ed. Walker D. Wyman and Clifton B. Kroeber (Madison: Univ. of Wisconsin Press, 1965), 59–77, A.L. Burt argues that conditions in New France generally had a "leveling influence" (64).

4. See also Richard Harrison Shryock, *Medical Licensing in America, 1650–1965* (Baltimore: Johns Hopkins Univ. Press, 1967), 9.

5. Previous estimates for the length of the medical apprenticeship have ranged from "typically three years" (Paul Starr), "generally from five to seven years" (Martin Kaufman), and "five to eight years" (Wyndham B. Blanton) to Lester S. King's simple statement that it was "long-term." Starr, *The Social Transformation of American Medicine* (New York: Basic Books, 1982), 40; Kaufman, *American Medical Education: The Formative Years, 1765–1910* (Westport, Conn.: Greenwood Press, 1976), 7; Blanton, *Medicine in Virginia in the Seventeenth Century* (Richmond: William Byrd Press, 1930), 97; King, "Medical Education: The Early Phases," *Journal of the American Medical Association* (1982), 48:731.

6. Daniel J. Boorstin, *The Americans: The Colonial Experience* (New York: Random House, 1958), 226; Raymond Phineas Stearns, *Science in the British Colonies of America* (Urbana: Univ. of Illinois Press, 1970), 417–18.

A Guide to Further Reading

There is no comprehensive history of medicine in the New World, although Francisco Guerra, "Medical Colonization of the New World," *Medical History* (1963), 7:147–54, provides a useful overview. Two works—P.M. Ashburn's older *The Ranks of Death: A Medical History of the Conquest of America* (New York: Coward-McCann, 1947) and Alfred W. Crosby's more recent *The Columbian Exchange: Biological and Cultural Consequences of 1492* (Westport, Conn.: Greenwood, 1972)—describe the medical effects of the European discovery of the New World, but both tend to emphasize developments in the Spanish colonies.

The best introduction to medicine in the British colonies is still found in Richard Harrison Shryock's brisk but perceptive survey of *Medicine and Society in America, 1660–1860* (New York: New York Univ. Press, 1960). The most extensive bibliography of medical literature in the British colonies appears in Francisco Guerra's *American Medical Bibliography, 1639–1783* (New York: L.C. Harper, 1962), but also see his "Medical Almanacs of the American Colonial Period," *Journal of the History of Medicine and Allied Sciences* (1961), 16:234–55.

In contrast to Edward Eggleston's pioneering study of *The Transit of Civilization from England to America in the Seventeenth Century* (New York: Appleton, 1901), which devotes a chapter to chronicling the decline of colonial medicine in the seventeenth century and generally avoids the issue of distinctive environmental influences, Daniel J. Boorstin's influential *The Americans: The Colonial Experience* (New York: Random House, 1958) contains a section on "New World

Medicine" that emphasizes the distinctiveness—and superiority—of medicine in the British colonies. Maurice Bear Gordon's detailed but old-fashioned *Aesculapius Comes to the Colonies: The Story of the Early Days of Medicine in the Thirteen Original Colonies* (Ventnor, N.J.: Ventnor Publishers, 1949) stresses the heroic and the biographical.

Among more specialized studies, John Duffy's *Epidemics in Colonial America* (Baton Rouge: Louisiana State Univ. Press, 1953) offers a comprehensive survey of colonial epidemics. In *Demography in Early America: Beginnings of the Statistical Mind, 1600–1800* (Cambridge, Mass.: Harvard Univ. Press, 1969) James H. Cassedy traces the growth of statistical methods, focusing particularly on their use in public health and medicine. Brooke Hindle's *The Pursuit of Science in Revolutionary America, 1735–1789* (Chapel Hill: Univ. of North Carolina Press, 1956), though featuring science more than medicine, devotes considerable attention to the cultivation of natural history by colonial physicians. Jane B. Donegan's *Women & Men Widwives: Medicine, Morality, and Misogyny in Early America* (Westport, Conn.: Greenwood Press, 1978) includes an extensive discussion of the colonial midwife and the growth of male midwifery in the eighteenth century.

THE MIDDLE ATLANTIC AND SOUTHERN COLONIES

Whitfield J. Bell, Jr., *The Colonial Physician and Other Essays* (New York: Science History Publications, 1975), a collection of previously published essays, sensitively explores medical life in colonial Philadelphia. His biography of *John Morgan: Continental Doctor* (Philadelphia: Univ. of Pennsylvania Press, 1965), who founded the first medical school in the English colonies, remains one of the best studies of a colonial physician. On Morgan's proposal to limit his practice to internal medicine, see Toby Gelfand, "The Origins of a Modern Concept of Medical Specialization: John Morgan's *Discourse* of 1765," *Bulletin of the History of Medicine* (1976), 50:511–35. For an introduction to Anglo-America's first permanent hospital, see William H. Williams, *America's First Hospital: The Pennsylvania Hospital, 1751–1841* (Wayne, Penn.: Haverford House, 1976). Various state and local histories of medicine devote a chapter or two to the colonial period; among the most useful accounts for the Middle Atlantic region are Part 1 of John Duffy's *A History of Public Health in New York City, 1625–1866* (New York: Russell Sage, 1968) and Chapter 1 of David L. Cowen's *Medicine and Health in New Jersey: A History* (Princeton, N.J.: D. Van Nostrand, 1964).

Wyndham B. Blanton's two fact-filled volumes on medicine in early Virginia—*Medicine in Virginia in the Seventeenth Century* (Richmond, Va.: William Byrd Press, 1930) and *Medicine in Virginia in the Eighteenth Century* (Richmond, Va.: Garrett & Massie, 1931)— are the starting point for any exploration of medicine in the colonial South. Also informative are Joseph Ioor Waring, *A History of Medicine in South Carolina, 1670–1825* (Columbia: South Carolina Medical Assoc., 1964), and John Duffy, ed., *The Rudolph Matas History of Medicine in Louisiana*, 2 vols. (Baton Rouge: Louisiana State Univ. Press, 1958), which includes coverage of Louisiana under the French and Spanish. The best biography of a southern colonial physician is Edmund Berkeley and Dorothy Smith Berkeley, *Dr. Alexander Garden of Charles Town* (Chapel Hill: Univ. of North Carolina Press, 1969).

Among the most valuable histories of disease and death in the colonial South are St. Julien Ravenel Childs, *Malaria and Colonization in the Carolina Low Country, 1526–1696* (Baltimore: Johns Hopkins Press, 1940); Darrett B. Rutman and Anita H. Rutman, "Of Agues and Fevers: Malaria in the Early Chesapeake," *William and Mary Quarterly*, 3rd ser. (1976), 33:31–60; and Carville V. Earle, "Environment, Disease, and Mortality in Early Virginia," in *The Chesapeake in the Seventeenth Century: Essays on Anglo-American Society*, ed. Thad W. Tate and David L. Ammerman (Chapel Hill: Univ. of North Carolina Press, 1979), 96–125.

OLD AND NEW ENGLAND

Excellent studies of medical practitioners in sixteenth- and seventeenth-century England include Margaret Pelling and Charles Webster, "Medical Practitioners," in *Health, Medicine and Mortality in the Sixteenth Century*, ed. Charles Webster (Cambridge: Cambridge Univ. Press, 1979), 165–235, Harold J. Cook, *The Decline of the Old Medical Regime in Stuart London* (Ithaca, N.Y.: Cornell Univ. Press, 1986); R.S. Roberts, "The Personnel and Practice of Medicine in Tudor and Stuart England," *Medical History* (1962), 6:363–82, and (1964), 8:217–34; Joseph F. Kett, "Provincial Medical Practice in England, 1730–1815," *Journal of the History of Medicine and Allied Sciences* (1964), 19:17–29; and Ronald C. Sawyer, "Patients, Healers, and Disease in the Southeast Midlands, 1597–1634" (Ph.D. diss., Univ. of Wisconsin-Madison, 1986).

The best comparable study for colonial New England is Philip J. Cash, Eric H. Christianson, and J. Worth Estes, eds., *Medicine in Colonial Massachusetts, 1620–1820*, vol. 57 of the *Publications of the Colonial Society of Massachusetts* (Boston: Colonial Society of Massachusetts, 1980), which includes essays on medical practitioners, the medical profession, and medical practice. A dated, but still useful, introduction that emphasizes the distinctiveness of colonial medicine is Malcolm Sydney Beinfield, "The Early New England Doctor: An Adaptation to a Provincial Environment," *Yale Journal of Biology and Medicine* (1942–43), *15*:99–132, 271–88. Particularly valuable for understanding the development of a profession of medicine are Eric H. Christianson, "The Emergence of Medical Communities in Massachusetts, 1700–1794: The Demographic Factors," *Bulletin of the History of Medicine* (1980), *54*:64–77; and Peter Dobkin Hall, "The Social Foundations of Professional Credibility: Linking the Medical Profession to Higher Education in Connecticut and Massachusetts, 1700–1830," in *The Authority of Experts: Studies in History and Theory,* ed. Thomas L. Haskell (Bloomington: Indiana Univ. Press, 1984), 107–41, which argues that "the early establishment of professional authority of a sort that far exceeded its clinical abilities was based precisely on [a] linkage of the profession to the college" (108).

In *Public Health in the Town of Boston, 1630–1822* (Cambridge, Mass.: Harvard Univ. Press, 1959) John B. Blake analyses the genesis of community public-health policies, which resulted in part from the threat of epidemics. One such outbreak of disease—attributable primarily to diphtheria—is described in Ernest Caulfield, "A True History of the Terrible Epidemic Vulgarly Called the Throat Distemper, Which Occurred in His Majesty's New England Colonies between the Years 1735 and 1740," *Yale Journal of Biology and Medicine* (1938–39), *11*:219–72, 277–335.

No person in the annals of colonial medical history has received more attention than the Reverend Cotton Mather, whose importance is reflected in the title of a biography by Otho T. Beall, Jr. and Richard H. Shryock, *Cotton Mather: First Significant Figure in American Medicine* (Baltimore: Johns Hopkins Press, 1954). Mather's previously unpublished *The Angel of Bethesda,* "the only systematic compilation of medical knowledge prepared in the English-American colonies," is now available in a version edited with introduction and notes by Gordon W. Jones (Barre, Mass.: American Antiquarian Society and Barre Publishers, 1972). Margaret Humphreys Warner offers a cogent analysis of the relationship between religion and medicine in Mather's writings in "Vindicating the Minister's Medical Role: Cotton Mather's Concept of the *Nishmath-Chajim* and the Spiritualization of Medicine," *Journal of the History of Medicine and Allied Sciences* (1981), *36*:278–95. For contrasting interpretations of Mather's involvement in the smallpox epidemic of 1721, see Ola Elizabeth Winslow's positive account in *A Destroying Angel: The Conquest of Smallpox in Colonial Boston* (Boston: Houghton Mifflin, 1974) and Perry Miller's critical assessment in his chapter on "The Judgment of Smallpox" in

The New England Mind: From Colony to Province (Boston: Beacon Press, 1953), 344–66. One of Mather's contemporaries, a preacher-physician named Thomas Palmer, has left a record of seventeenth-century medical practice in his commonplace book, completed in 1696 and recently published under the title *The Admirable Secrets of Physick and Chyrurgery,* ed. Thomas Rogers Forbes (New Haven: Yale Univ. Press, 1984).

Two illuminating studies of medicine in New England during the time of the Revolutionary War are J. Worth Estes, *Hall Jackson and the Purple Foxglove: Medical Practice & Research in Revolutionary America, 1760–1820* (Hanover, N.H.: Univ. Press of New England), which features the physician who introduced digitalis into American medical practice; and Philip Cash, *Medical Men at the Siege of Boston, April, 1775–April, 1776: Problems of the Massachusetts and Continental Armies* (Philadelphia: American Philosophical Society, 1973), which describes not only the care of the sick but also the logistical problems that faced military doctors.

OLD AND NEW SPAIN

There is no adequate introduction in English to the history of Spanish medicine, although a skeleton is provided by Fielding H. Garrison, "An Epitome of the History of Spanish Medicine," *Bulletin of the New York Academy of Medicine* (1931), 7:589–634. For a convenient survey in Spanish of developments in the sixteenth and seventeenth centuries, see chapters 2 and 3 of Luis S. Granjel, *Historia de la medicina española* (Barcelona: Sayma, 1962). Two useful bibliographical guides are Antonio Hernández Morejón, *Historia bibliográfica de la medicina española,* originally published in Madrid in 1842–1845 and reprinted in 7 vols. in 1967, with an introduction by Francisco Guerra (New York: Johnson Reprint Corp.); and Luis S. Granjel, *Bibliografía histórica de la medicina española,* 2 vols. (Salmanca: Univ. of Salamanca, 1957, 1966).

For background regarding the history of New Spain, the following works are recommended: Daniel Cosio Villegas and others, *A Compact History of Mexico,* trans. Marjory Mattingly Urquidi (México: El Colegio de México, 1974); Henry B. Parkes, *A History of Mexico* (Boston: Houghton Mifflin, 1970), a popular text; Murdo J. MacLeod, *Spanish Central America: A Socio-Economic History, 1520–1720* (Berkeley: Univ. of California Press, 1973); and Peggy K. Liss, *Mexico under Spain, 1521–1556* (Chicago: Univ. of Chicago Press, 1975), which analyzes early social changes. The fate of the Indians is discussed by

Charles Gibson in *The Aztecs under Spanish Rule* (Stanford, Calif.: Stanford Univ. Press, 1964), while Peter Gerhard's *A Guide to the Historical Geography of New Spain* (Cambridge: Cambridge Univ. Press, 1972) provides a detailed region-by-region analysis. For additional references, consult Edna M. Orozco and Alma R. Platus, eds., *Bibliografía general de la historia de Mexico* (México: Instituto Nacional de Antropologia e Historia, 1979).

The history of medicine in New Spain remains largely unwritten, although the recently published study of *The Royal Protomedicato: The Regulation of the Medical Professions in the Spanish Empire* (Durham, N.C.: Duke Univ. Press, 1985), written by the late John Tate Lanning and edited by John Jay TePaske, fills a large void. Two earlier studies by Lanning—*Academic Culture in the Spanish Colonies* (London: Oxford Univ. Press, 1940), which devotes two chapters to medical matters, and *Pedro de la Torre: Doctor to Conquerors* (Baton Rouge: Louisiana State Univ. Press, 1974), a biography of a mid-sixteenth-century practitioner in New Spain—are also valuable contributions to the literature.

The Mexican National Academy of Medicine, under the direction of Fernando Martínez Cortés, has undertaken an ambitious multivolume survey of Mexican medicine from prehistorical times to the present, the first volumes of which will soon appear. In the meantime, we must rely on such works as Francisco A. Flores's outdated but still useful *Historia de la medicina en México desde la epoca de los Indios hasta la presente,* 3 vols. (México: Secretaría de Fomento, 1886–88), and Josefina Muriel's *Hospitales de la Nueva España,* 2 vols. (México: Publicaciones del Instituto de Historia, 1956, and Editorial Jus. Mexico, 1960). Gordon Schendel's popular *Medicine in Mexico* (Austin: Univ. of Texas Press, 1968) includes several chapters on the colonial period, as does John Z. Bowers and Elizabeth F. Purcell, eds., *Aspects of the History of Medicine in Latin America* (New York: Josiah Macy, Jr. Foundation, 1979). Helpful information can also be gleaned from E.E. Hume, "Spanish Colonial Medicine," *Bulletin of the Institute of the History of Medicine* (1934), 2:125–30, and Saul Jarcho, "Medicine in Sixteenth Century New Spain as Illustrated by the Writings of Bravo, Farfan, and Vargas Machuca," *Bulletin of the History of Medicine* (1957), 31:425–41.

Francisco Guerra discusses the history of medical practice and drug therapy in *Historia de la materia médica Hispanoamericana e Filipina en la epoca colonial* (Madrid: A. Aguado, 1973). Guenter B. Risse's "Transcending Cultural Barriers: The European Reception of Medicinal Plants from the Americas," in *Botanical Drugs of the Americas in the Old and New Worlds,* ed. Wolfgang-Hagen Hein (Stuttgart: Wissenschaftliche Verlagsgesellschaft MBH, 1984), 31–42, focuses on the European assimilation of drugs from New Spain in the sixteenth century. For a guide to the pharmaceutical literature, see G. Simmons Gittinger, "A Selected Bibliography of Pharmacy in Latin America," *American Journal of Pharmaceutical Education* (1959), 23:424–29.

The late Germán Somolinos D'Ardois wrote four small volumes on the history of medicine in New Spain, all published by the Mexican Society of the History and Philosophy of Medicine as part of its series *Capitulos de historia médica Mexicana*. The first, *Medicina en las culturas Mesoamericanas anteriores a la conquista* (1978), looks at pre-Columbian healing practices. The second, *El fenómeno de fusión cultural y su trascendencia médica* (1979), discusses the effects of Spanish acculturation and the use of native herbs. The third, *Relación alfabética de los profesionalistas médicos, 1521–1618* (1980), contains biographical sketches of health professionals prominent in New Spain during its first century. The fourth, *Relación y estudio de los impresos médicos Mexicanos redactados y editados desde 1521 a 1618* (1981), offers a chronological analysis of the medical literature in the same period.

There are several useful bibliographies relating to medicine in New Spain. Joaquín García Icazbalceta's classic *Bibliografía Mexicana del siglo XVI* (México: Fondo de Cultura Económica, 1954) devotes a section to medicine titled "Los médicos de México en el siglo XVI" (222–42). Francisco Guerra has prepared a more recent guide covering all the Latin American colonies—*Historiografía de la medicina colonial Hispanoamericana* (México: Abastecedora de Impresos, 1953)—as well as a separate bibliography specifically on Mexican medicine: "La bibliografía de historia de la medicina Mexicana," *La Prensa Médica Mexicana (1949)*, 14:87–93. M.T. Esquivel Olea identifies the medical collections in the National Archives of Mexico that deal with hospitals and the *protomedicato* in *Indice de los ramos hospitales y protomedicato* (México: Archivo General de la Nación, 1977) For hospitals, see also D.B. Cooper, "A Selective List of the Colonial Manuscripts (1564–1800) in the Archives of the Department of Health and Welfare, Mexico City: A Newly Discovered Source for Religious and Architectural History," *Hispanic America Historical Review* (1967), 18:385–414.

OLD AND NEW FRANCE

In recent years the history of medicine in early modern France has attracted considerable attention. Studies by historians of the *Annales* school of Paris have resulted in two important collections of essays in English translation, both edited by Robert Forster and Orest Ranum and translated by Elborg Forster and Patricia M. Ranum: *Biology of Man in History: Selections from the Annales: Economies, Sociétés, Civilisations* (Baltimore: Johns Hopkins Univ. Press, 1975), which includes essays on the history of disease; and *Medicine and Society in France: Selections from the Annales: Economiés, Sociétés, Civilisations* (Baltimore: Johns Hopkins Univ. Press, 1980), which looks at the medical profession. Important recent monographs in English dealing with the medical and surgical professions and public health in Old Regime France are Toby Gelfand, *Professionalizing Modern Medicine: Paris Surgeons and Medical Science and Institutions in the 18th Century* (Westport, Conn.: Greenwood Press, 1980); Caroline C. Hannaway, "Medicine, Public Welfare, and the State in Eighteenth-Century France: The Société Royale de Médecine (1776–1793)" (unpubl. Ph.D. diss., Johns Hopkins Univ., 1974); and Matthew Ramsey, *Professional and Popular Medicine in France, 1770–1830: The Social World of Medical Practice* (Cambridge: Cambridge Univ. Press, 1987). Also valuable are the French studies by Paul Delaunay, *La vie médicale aux XVIe, XVIIe et XVIIIe siècles* (Paris: Hippocrate, 1935); François Lebrun, *Les hommes et la mort en Anjou au XVIIe siècles* (Paris: Mouton, 1971); and Jean-Pierre Goubert, *Malades et médecins en Bretagne, 1770–1790* (Paris: Klincksieck, 1974).

The secondary literature on medicine in New France is much scanter, older, and less critical, and relatively little is available in English. Marcel Trudel's *Initiation à la Nouvelle France* (Montreal: Holt, Rinehart et Winston, 1968), which appeared in English translation under the title *Introduction to New France* (Toronto: Holt, Rinehart, and Winston, 1968), provides the best concise survey of the subject and points out the need for additional research in the history of public health and medicine in New France. To some extent, the first four volumes of the *Dictionary of Canadian Biography* (1966–1979), edited by George W. Brown and published jointly by the University of Toronto Press and Presses de l'Université Laval in Quebec, have responded to this need. These volumes, which cover persons who died before 1801, contain some fifty sketches of medical men in New France that often make extensive use of archival materials. For an analysis of this small but revealing sample, see Toby Gelfand, "Who Practiced Medicine in New France? A Collective Portrait," in *Health, Disease and Medicine: Essays in Canadian History*, ed. Charles Roland (Toronto: Clarke Irwin, 1984), 16–35. The civil, military, and religious archives of the mother country await systematic exploration for documents relating to medicine in New France.

Despite its biographical approach, Arthur Vallée, *Un biologiste Canadien, Michel Sarrazin, 1659–1735: Sa vie, ses travaux et son temps*

(Quebec: Imprimerie du roi, 1927), offers a broad survey of medicine in New France. Other useful secondary sources include Mary Loretto Gies, *Mère Duplessis de Sainte Hélène, annaliste et epistolière* (unpublished *thèse de doctorat*, Université Laval, 1949); Maud E. Abbot, *History of Medicine in the Province of Quebec* (Montreal: McGill, 1931); and J.J. Heagerty, *Four Centuries of Medical History in Canada* (Toronto: Macmillan, 1928).

The best summary of the medical profession and medical institutions in New France is Gabriel Nadeau, "Le dernier chirurgien du roi à Québec: Antoine Briault, 1742–1760," *L'Union Médicale du Canada* (1951), 80:705–26. Other useful accounts of medical practitioners, which tend to be annotated lists, include M.-J. and Georges Ahern, *Notes pour servir à l'histoire de la médecine dans le Bas-Canada, depuis la fondation de Quebec jusqu'au commencement du XIXᵉ siècle* (Quebec, 1923); E.-Z. Massicotte, "Les chirurgiens, médecins, etc., etc., de Montréal sous le régime français," *Rapport de l'Archiviste du Province de Québec* (1922–23), 3:131–55, and several other follow-up articles by the same author in *Bulletin des Recherches Historiques;* Raymond Douville, "Chirurgiens, barbiers-chirurgiens et charlatans de la région trifluvienne sous le régime francais," *Cahiers de Dix* (1950), 15:81–128. The anthology *Trois siècles de médecine québecoise* (Québec: La Société Historique de Québec, 1970) contains articles on medicine in New France by Sylvio Leblond and Antonio Drolet. François Rousseau's "Hôpital et société en Nouvelle France: L'Hôtel-Dieu de Québec à la fin du XVIIᵉ siècle," *Revue d'Histoire de l'Amérique Française* (1977), 31:29–47, is a critical quantitative study based on the author's 1974 master's thesis at Université Laval.

For a thorough discussion of military medicine during the War of Conquest, see Jean des Cilleuls, "L'Oeuvre du service de santé au cours de la guerre de 1755–1760," *Histoire de la Médecine* (May 1960), 10:8–55. On midwives, see Hélène Laforce, *Histoire de la sage-femme dans la région de Québec* (Québec: Institut Québécois de Recherche sur la Culture, 1985). Very little has been published on the history of diseases and public health in New France, but a search of the periodical literature, especially the *Bulletin des Recherches Historiques* and the *Rapport de L'Archiviste du Province de Québec*, will yield many brief accounts on these and related subjects as well as some pertinent original documents.

Contributors

ERIC II. CHRISTIANSON is Associate Professor of History at the University of Kentucky, where he has taught since 1975. As a graduate student in history, he studied at the University of Cambridge and at the University of Southern California, where he received a Ph.D. degree in 1976. In addition to co-editing *Medicine in Colonial Massachusetts, 1630-1820* (1980), he has written a number of articles on science and medicine in early America. He is currently writing a book on science and medicine at Transylvania University.

TOBY GELFAND is Jason A. Hannah Professor of the History of Medicine at the University of Ottawa. After studying medicine for three years at the University of Pennsylvania, he enrolled in the Johns Hopkins Institute of the History of Medicine, which awarded him a Ph.D. degree in 1973. His publications include *Professionalizing Modern Medicine: Paris Surgeons and Medical Science and Institutions in the 18th Century* (1980) and many articles on eighteenth-century medicine in Europe and North America. He is currently working on a study of "Medical Discourse and the Jews in France (1850-1900)."

RONALD L. NUMBERS is Professor of the History of Medicine and the History of Science at the University of Wisconsin-

Madison. A graduate of the University of California at Berkeley (Ph.D., 1969), he has written or edited a number of books, including *Prophetess of Health: A Study of Ellen G. White* (1976) and *Almost Persuaded: American Physicians and Compulsory Health Insurance, 1912-1920* (1978). His current research focuses on the history of "scientific creationism" in the twentieth century, for which he received a fellowship from the John Simon Guggenheim Memorial Foundation.

GUENTER B. RISSE is Professor and Chairman, Department of the History and Philosophy of Health Sciences, University of California, San Francisco. He received his medical training at the University of Buenos Aires (M.D., 1958) and his historical training at the University of Chicago (Ph.D., 1971). He is the author of *Hospital Life in Enlightenment Scotland: Care and Teaching at the Royal Infirmary of Edinburgh* (1986), as well as dozens of articles on the history of medicine, from antiquity to the present. He is currently completing a study of Brunonianism in Europe and America.

Index*

---

*Prepared by Charlotte Borst

This book was designed by Sheila Hart; composed by Lithocraft, Inc., Grundy Center, Iowa; printed by Thomson-Shore, Inc., Dexter, Michigan; and bound by John H. Dekker & Sons, Grand Rapids, Michigan. The book was set in 10/12 Sabon display and printed on 60-lb. Warren's Olde Style wove.

THE UNIVERSITY OF TENNESSEE PRESS